**Daily Ayurveda:
Ancient Wisdom for Modern Living**

By Bhuvanyu Singh

List of Chapters:

Part 1: Understanding Ayurveda

1. **Introduction to Ayurveda**
   - History and Philosophy
   - The Three Doshas: Vata, Pitta, and Kapha
   - The Concept of Prakriti (Constitution)
2. **The Science of Doshas**
   - Characteristics of Each Dosha
   - Identifying Your Dominant Dosha
   - Balancing Doshas in Daily Life

Part 2: Daily Ayurvedic Practices

1. **Morning Routines for Wellness**
   - Dinacharya: The Ayurvedic Daily Routine
   - Morning Practices: Tongue Scraping, Oil Pulling, and Abhyanga (Self-Massage)
   - Ayurvedic Breakfasts
2. **Ayurvedic Nutrition**
   - The Six Tastes in Ayurveda
   - Eating for Your Dosha
   - Seasonal Eating
3. **Midday Practices for Energy**
   - Ayurvedic Lunch Tips
   - Importance of Agni (Digestive Fire)
   - Herbal Teas and Remedies
4. **Evening Routines for Rest**
   - Calming Practices Before Bed
   - Ayurvedic Dinners
   - Sleep Hygiene

Part 3: Mind, Body, and Spirit

1. **Mindful Movement**
   - Yoga for Your Dosha
   - Pranayama (Breathing Exercises)
   - Meditation Techniques
2. **Ayurvedic Self-Care**
   - Skin and Hair Care Routines
   - Ayurvedic Beauty Secrets
   - Self-Massage Techniques
3. **Ayurvedic Healing**
   - Common Ayurvedic Remedies
   - Detoxification and Panchakarma
   - Managing Stress and Anxiety
4. **Seasonal Ayurveda**
   - Adapting Practices with the Seasons
   - Seasonal Diet and Lifestyle Tips
   - Staying Balanced Year-Round

Part 4: Special Topics

1. **Ayurveda for Families**
   - Ayurvedic Practices for Children
   - Family Meals and Routines
   - Teaching Ayurveda to Kids
2. **Ayurveda in the Workplace**
   - Staying Balanced at Work
   - Ayurvedic Tips for Office Life
   - Managing Work Stress
3. **Ayurvedic Travel Tips**
   - Staying Balanced on the Go
   - Travel-Friendly Ayurvedic Practices
   - Adapting Your Routine

Part 5: Deepening Your Practice

1. **Advanced Ayurvedic Techniques**

    - Rasayana (Rejuvenation Therapy)
    - Advanced Herbal Treatments
    - Deeper Detox Practices
2. **Integrating Ayurveda with Other Practices**
    - Combining Ayurveda with Modern Medicine
    - Integrating Other Holistic Practices
    - Building a Comprehensive Wellness Plan
3. **Conclusion: Embracing Ayurveda**
    - Sustaining Your Ayurvedic Lifestyle
    - Continuing Education and Resources
    - Community and Support

Introduction:

In today's fast-paced world, where stress is prevalent and balance seems elusive, the ancient wisdom of Ayurveda offers a beacon of hope. Rooted in the timeless principles of holistic health, Ayurveda provides a comprehensive framework for harmonizing mind, body, and spirit. In "Daily Ayurveda: Ancient Wisdom for Modern Living," we embark on a journey to rediscover this profound tradition and integrate its practices into our daily lives.

Part 1 serves as our gateway into the world of Ayurveda, where we explore its history, philosophy, and fundamental principles. Central to Ayurveda are the three doshas - Vata, Pitta, and Kapha - dynamic forces that govern our unique constitution, or Prakriti. By understanding the interplay of these doshas within ourselves, we gain insight into our individual needs and how to achieve balance.

Moving into Part 2, we delve into practical applications of Ayurveda for daily living. From morning rituals to evening routines, we learn how to align our lifestyle with the natural rhythms of the day. Discover the art of Ayurvedic nutrition, incorporating the six tastes to nourish our bodies according to their inherent needs. Harness the power of herbal remedies and teas to support digestion, vitality, and overall well-being.

Part 3 explores the holistic nature of Ayurveda, encompassing practices for nurturing the mind, body, and spirit. Engage in mindful movement with dosha-specific yoga practices, and explore the transformative effects of pranayama and meditation. Embrace self-care rituals, from skincare to rejuvenating self-massage techniques, and discover Ayurvedic remedies for common ailments and stress management.

In Part 4, we delve into specialized topics, offering guidance on incorporating Ayurveda into family life, the workplace, and travel. Learn how to adapt Ayurvedic principles to meet the needs of your family, cultivate balance amidst the demands of work, and maintain wellness on the go. Embrace the changing seasons with practices tailored to support your well-being year-round.

Finally, Part 5 offers insights into advanced Ayurvedic techniques and strategies for integrating Ayurveda with other wellness modalities. Explore the intersection of Ayurveda and modern medicine, and develop a personalized wellness plan that honors your unique needs and goals.

As we embark on this journey together, may the wisdom of Ayurveda illuminate our path to vibrant health and profound well-being. Let us embrace this ancient tradition with gratitude and reverence, knowing that each step we take brings us closer to a life of balance, harmony, and fulfilment.

Part 1: Understanding Ayurveda

History and Philosophy

Ayurveda, often translated as the "science of life," is one of the world's oldest holistic healing systems. Its origins can be traced back more than 5,000 years to the Indian subcontinent, where it was developed through a profound understanding of the laws of nature and the intricate workings of the human body and mind. This ancient system of medicine is based on the belief that health and wellness depend on a delicate balance between the mind, body, and spirit. The primary goal of Ayurveda is to promote good health, not just to fight disease.

The history of Ayurveda is deeply intertwined with the spiritual and philosophical traditions of India. It is said to have been divinely revealed to the ancient sages, or rishis, who were the first to practice and codify this knowledge. These sages were deeply connected to nature and observed the effects of various natural substances on the human body. Through meditation and introspection, they developed a comprehensive system of health and healing that addressed all aspects of life.

One of the foundational texts of Ayurveda is the "Charaka Samhita," attributed to the sage Charaka, which focuses on the diagnosis and treatment of diseases. Another key text is the "Sushruta Samhita," attributed to the sage Sushruta, which is renowned for its detailed descriptions of surgical techniques and procedures. These ancient texts, written in Sanskrit, are still revered today and provide a vast repository of medical knowledge.

Ayurveda is built upon a unique philosophy that views the universe and everything in it, including the human body, as composed of five fundamental elements: earth, water, fire, air, and ether (space). These elements combine to form three primary life forces or doshas: Vata, Pitta, and Kapha. Each dosha represents a different combination of elements and governs specific physiological and psychological functions in the body.

Vata, composed of air and ether, is associated with movement and change. It governs all bodily functions related to motion, such as breathing, circulation, and nerve impulses. Individuals with a predominant Vata dosha are often energetic, creative, and quick-thinking but may also be prone to anxiety, restlessness, and digestive issues when out of balance.

Pitta, made up of fire and water, is linked to transformation and metabolism. It controls the body's metabolic processes, including digestion, absorption, and temperature regulation. People with a dominant Pitta dosha tend to be intelligent, ambitious, and determined but can experience irritability, inflammation, and overheating if their Pitta is imbalanced.

Kapha, consisting of earth and water, is connected to structure and stability. It oversees the body's growth, tissue formation, and immune function. Those with a predominant Kapha dosha are generally calm, compassionate, and strong but may struggle with weight gain, congestion, and lethargy when Kapha is excessive.

The balance of these doshas is crucial for maintaining health. Each person's unique combination of Vata, Pitta, and Kapha is referred to as their prakriti, or constitution, which is determined at the moment of conception and remains constant throughout life. However, various factors such as diet, lifestyle, stress, and environmental conditions can disturb this balance, leading to vikriti, or imbalance, which can manifest as physical or mental illness.

Ayurveda emphasizes the importance of living in harmony with nature's cycles and rhythms to maintain doshic balance. This includes following a daily routine (dinacharya) that aligns with the natural world, such as waking up early, eating meals at regular times, and getting adequate rest. Seasonal routines (ritucharya) are also recommended to adjust one's lifestyle and diet according to the changing seasons.

Diet and nutrition play a central role in Ayurveda. Food is considered medicine, and each meal is an opportunity to balance the doshas. Ayurvedic dietary guidelines take into account an individual's prakriti, the properties of different foods, and how they interact with the doshas. For instance, a Vata-balancing diet might include warm, moist, and grounding foods, while a Pitta-balancing diet might focus on cooling and calming foods.

In addition to diet, Ayurveda incorporates a variety of therapeutic practices to restore balance and promote healing. These include herbal medicine, yoga, meditation, massage (abhyanga), detoxification (panchakarma), and breathing exercises (pranayama). Each treatment is tailored to the individual's unique constitution and specific imbalances.

The philosophy of Ayurveda also extends to the mind and spirit. It recognizes the profound connection between mental and physical health and emphasizes the importance of mental well-being. Practices such as meditation, mindfulness, and self-inquiry are integral to maintaining mental balance and achieving a state of inner peace.

In essence, Ayurveda offers a holistic approach to health and wellness that is deeply rooted in the understanding of the interconnectedness of all life. Its time-tested principles and practices provide a comprehensive framework for living a balanced and harmonious life. By understanding and applying the wisdom of Ayurveda, individuals can cultivate a deeper awareness of their own unique constitution, make informed choices about their health, and embark on a journey of self-discovery and healing.

The Three Doshas:

Vata, Pitta, and Kapha

In the heart of Ayurveda lies the concept of the three doshas: Vata, Pitta, and Kapha. These doshas are the fundamental bioenergies that govern the physical and mental processes of the human body and mind. Derived from the five elements (earth, water, fire, air, and ether), the doshas form the foundation for understanding individual constitution, health, and disease in Ayurvedic medicine. Each person has a unique combination of these doshas, which determines their prakriti, or natural constitution, and influences their physiological and psychological traits.

Vata, the first of the three doshas, is composed of air and ether. It is the principle of movement and is responsible for all bodily functions related to motion, including breathing, circulation, and the transmission of nerve impulses. Vata governs the energy of movement and is often described as dry, light, cold, rough, subtle, and mobile. Individuals with a dominant Vata dosha tend to be energetic, creative, and quick-thinking. They are often slender with dry skin and cold hands and feet. When balanced, Vata types are lively, enthusiastic, and adaptable. However, when out of balance, they may experience anxiety, restlessness, insomnia, and digestive issues such as bloating and constipation.

To maintain balance, Vata individuals benefit from routines that provide stability and warmth. They should favor warm, cooked foods that are moist and nourishing, such as soups, stews, and porridges. Regular meals, adequate rest, and gentle exercises like yoga and walking are also beneficial. Additionally, practices that promote grounding and relaxation, such as meditation and oil massage (abhyanga), help to soothe the mobile and erratic nature of Vata.

Pitta, the second dosha, is made up of fire and water. It embodies the principle of transformation and is responsible for the body's metabolic processes, including digestion, absorption, and temperature regulation. Pitta is characterized by qualities such as hot, sharp, light, oily, and intense. Those with a predominant Pitta dosha typically have a medium build, warm body temperature, and strong appetite. They are known for their intelligence, ambition, and leadership qualities. When balanced, Pitta individuals are focused, perceptive, and courageous. However, an imbalance can lead to irritability, anger, inflammation, and digestive issues like heartburn and acid reflux.

To keep Pitta in check, individuals should seek cooling and soothing influences. This includes consuming foods that are sweet, bitter, and astringent, such as leafy greens, melons, and dairy products. It is also important for Pitta types to avoid excessive heat and to engage in calming activities that reduce stress, such as swimming, nature walks, and mindfulness practices. Incorporating relaxation techniques and ensuring adequate hydration are key to maintaining Pitta balance.

Kapha, the third dosha, is composed of earth and water. It is the energy of structure and stability, providing the body with strength, cohesion, and lubrication. Kapha is described as heavy, slow, steady, solid, cold, soft, and oily. Individuals with a dominant Kapha dosha often have a sturdy build, smooth skin, and a calm demeanor. They are known for their endurance, loyalty, and compassionate nature. When in balance, Kapha individuals are strong, nurturing, and patient. However, an imbalance can result in weight gain, lethargy, depression, and congestion.

To balance Kapha, it is essential to incorporate stimulating and invigorating practices into daily life. This includes consuming light, dry, and warming foods, such as spices, legumes, and green vegetables. Regular physical activity, especially vigorous exercise, is crucial to counteract Kapha's natural tendency towards inertia. Additionally, activities that promote mental and emotional stimulation, such as social interactions and creative pursuits, can help to keep Kapha balanced and vibrant.

Understanding the interplay of the three doshas is fundamental to the practice of Ayurveda. Each dosha not only governs specific physiological and psychological functions but also interacts with the others to maintain overall health and balance. This dynamic relationship is evident in every aspect of life, from digestion and metabolism to emotions and behavior.

Ayurveda teaches that the key to health lies in recognizing and honoring one's unique doshic constitution while adapting lifestyle and dietary habits to maintain balance. This personalized approach to wellness allows individuals to prevent illness, promote longevity, and achieve a state of harmony with the natural world.

In essence, Vata, Pitta, and Kapha offer a comprehensive framework for understanding the complexities of human health and behavior. By embracing the principles of Ayurveda and integrating them into daily life, individuals can cultivate a deeper awareness of their own bodies and minds, leading to a more balanced, fulfilling, and harmonious existence.

The Concept of Prakriti (Constitution)

The concept of Prakriti, or constitution, is fundamental to understanding Ayurveda, the ancient Indian system of holistic medicine. Prakriti refers to an individual's unique physical and psychological constitution, which is determined at the time of conception. This innate constitution is influenced by the combination of the three doshas—Vata, Pitta, and Kapha—present at the moment of one's birth. Prakriti remains unchanged throughout a person's life and governs their tendencies, strengths, and susceptibilities.

Each person's Prakriti is a unique blend of the three doshas, with one or two usually being more dominant. This specific combination of doshas influences an individual's physical characteristics, mental and emotional tendencies, and overall health. Understanding one's Prakriti provides a roadmap for maintaining balance and preventing disease.

The assessment of Prakriti involves a detailed analysis of various physical, mental, and emotional traits. This includes examining body type, skin texture, hair type, digestion, metabolism, temperament, and emotional responses. Practitioners of Ayurveda use these observations to determine the dominant doshas and thereby identify the Prakriti.

Individuals with a Vata-dominant Prakriti tend to have a light, slender body frame with dry skin and cold extremities. They are often energetic, creative, and quick learners but may struggle with anxiety, restlessness, and irregular sleep patterns. Their digestion can be variable, and they might experience bloating and constipation.

Those with a Pitta-dominant Prakriti generally have a medium build, warm skin, and a strong appetite. They are intelligent, focused, and often exhibit strong leadership qualities. However, they may be prone to irritability, impatience, and inflammatory conditions such as heartburn or skin rashes. Pitta individuals typically have a robust digestive system but can suffer from acidity and heat-related issues if out of balance.

Kapha-dominant individuals usually have a larger, well-built frame with smooth, oily skin and thick hair. They are known for their calm, steady, and compassionate nature, but can become lethargic, resistant to change, and prone to weight gain. Their digestion is slow and steady, and they are more susceptible to conditions involving mucus and congestion.

Understanding Prakriti extends beyond merely categorizing body types. It encompasses a holistic view of health, emphasizing the importance of maintaining the natural balance of the doshas to prevent disease. Ayurveda teaches that health is not a one-size-fits-all approach but rather a personalized practice that considers individual differences in constitution.

Prakriti influences dietary needs, lifestyle choices, exercise preferences, and even suitable daily routines. For instance, a Vata-dominant person may benefit from a warm, grounding diet that includes cooked vegetables, grains, and warm spices, along with a regular routine that emphasizes stability and rest. In contrast, a Pitta-dominant individual might thrive on cooling foods like fresh fruits and vegetables, avoiding overly spicy or sour foods, and incorporating relaxation techniques to manage stress.

Kapha-dominant individuals may need a stimulating and light diet, including spicy and bitter foods, and an active lifestyle to counteract their natural tendency towards sluggishness. They should engage in vigorous exercise and avoid heavy, oily foods that can exacerbate Kapha imbalance.

In addition to dietary and lifestyle recommendations, Ayurveda offers various treatments tailored to an individual's Prakriti. These may include herbal remedies, detoxification processes like Panchakarma, and specific yoga and meditation practices designed to balance the doshas.

The concept of Prakriti also underscores the importance of self-awareness and self-care in Ayurvedic philosophy. By understanding their unique constitution, individuals can make informed choices that align with their natural tendencies, promoting long-term health and well-being. This personalized approach to health helps prevent disease by addressing imbalances before they manifest as illness.

Moreover, Prakriti influences psychological traits and emotional health. Vata types may need practices that calm the mind and reduce anxiety, such as grounding yoga poses and meditation. Pitta types benefit from activities that cool the mind and body, like swimming or mindfulness meditation, to prevent stress and anger. Kapha types may require stimulating activities that invigorate the mind and body, such as dynamic yoga and active hobbies, to ward off depression and lethargy.

The interplay between Prakriti and lifestyle is dynamic and requires ongoing attention. Seasonal changes, environmental factors, and life stages can all impact the balance of doshas. For example, the Vata season (fall and early winter) might exacerbate Vata qualities, necessitating additional measures to stay grounded and warm. Similarly, the hot, dry conditions of the Pitta season (summer) require cooling and hydrating practices to keep Pitta in check.

Ayurveda also recognizes the concept of Vikriti, which refers to the current state of imbalance in the doshas. While Prakriti is constant, Vikriti fluctuates based on lifestyle, diet, stress, and other factors. Ayurvedic practitioners assess both Prakriti and Vikriti to provide comprehensive guidance aimed at restoring balance and promoting optimal health.

In essence, the concept of Prakriti in Ayurveda offers a profound understanding of individual health and well-being. It emphasizes that health is a personalized journey, deeply rooted in understanding and aligning with one's natural constitution. By embracing this holistic perspective, individuals can achieve a harmonious balance of body, mind, and spirit, leading to a more fulfilling and healthy life.

2. The Science of Doshas

Characteristics of Each Dosha

Vata

Understanding Vata

In the rich tapestry of Ayurvedic philosophy, the dosha known as Vata is revered as the dynamic force that governs movement, creativity, and change within the human body and mind. Derived from the elemental energies of air and ether, Vata orchestrates the subtle rhythms of existence, shaping our individuality and influencing our interactions with the world around us.

The Essence of Vata

Vata, with its ethereal essence, embodies the very essence of movement and transformation. Much like the wind that dances through the trees or the flowing currents of a river, Vata pervades every aspect of our being, propelling us forward on the journey of life. Individuals with a predominant Vata constitution are often described as lively, imaginative, and spontaneous, with a natural inclination towards exploration and innovation.

Physical Characteristics

In the realm of the physical body, Vata manifests itself through a delicate interplay of qualities that reflect its elemental nature. Vata types typically exhibit a slender, wiry physique, with long limbs and graceful movements that echo the fluidity of the wind. Their features are often characterized by sharp angles and fine bone structure, lending an air of ethereal elegance to their appearance. Yet, beneath this surface, Vata individuals may also experience tendencies towards dryness and variability, with skin that is prone to dryness and hair that is fine and brittle.

Mental and Emotional Traits

The influence of Vata extends far beyond the realm of the physical, shaping the landscape of the mind and emotions with its boundless energy and creativity. Vata types possess a keen intellect and a quick wit, with minds that are constantly in motion, exploring new ideas and seeking out novel experiences. They are natural-born communicators, adept at expressing themselves through words, art, or music, and thrive in environments that allow for freedom of expression and exploration.

However, the same qualities that make Vata types so vibrant and dynamic can also leave them susceptible to imbalances when in excess. In times of stress or upheaval, Vata individuals may experience feelings of anxiety, fear, or restlessness, as their minds spin with a whirlwind of thoughts and emotions. Learning to cultivate grounding practices and establish a sense of stability can be essential for restoring balance and harmony within the Vata dosha.

Balancing Vata

In Ayurveda, maintaining balance within the Vata dosha is seen as crucial for supporting overall health and well-being. This may involve incorporating grounding and nourishing practices into daily life, such as establishing a regular routine, engaging in gentle exercise like yoga or tai chi, and prioritizing warm, moist, and grounding foods in the diet. By honoring the unique qualities of Vata and embracing practices that promote balance and stability, individuals can harness the transformative power of this ancient wisdom, leading to a life filled with vitality, creativity, and fulfillment.

As we journey through the intricate landscape of Ayurvedic wisdom, the dosha of Vata emerges as a dynamic force of energy and movement, guiding us towards greater understanding and self-awareness. By cultivating an awareness of our individual Vata constitution and embracing practices that foster balance and stability, we can unlock the full potential of this ancient wisdom, leading to a life filled with vitality, creativity, and fulfillment.

Pitta

Understanding Pitta

In the intricate tapestry of Ayurveda, the dosha known as Pitta emerges as a fiery force of transformation, embodying the qualities of intensity, intelligence, and ambition. Comprised of the elemental energies of fire and water, Pitta governs the subtle rhythms of digestion, metabolism, and vitality within the human body and mind, shaping our experiences of health, temperament, and interaction with the world.

The Essence of Pitta

Pitta, with its fiery nature, serves as the driving force behind the processes of transformation and metabolism within the body. Much like the flames that dance in the hearth, Pitta imbues us with a sense of warmth, energy, and vitality, propelling us forward on the journey of life. Individuals with a predominant Pitta constitution are often described as ambitious, focused, and driven, possessing a natural inclination towards leadership and achievement.

Physical Characteristics

Physically, Pitta manifests itself through a unique interplay of qualities that reflect its elemental composition. Pitta types typically exhibit a medium build, with strong musculature and a sharp, penetrating gaze that reflects their intense energy and determination. Their features are often characterized by a symmetrical appearance, with well-defined jawlines and piercing eyes that exude confidence and charisma. Yet, beneath this surface, Pitta individuals may also experience tendencies towards heat and inflammation, with skin that is prone to sensitivity and irritation.

Mental and Emotional Traits

The influence of Pitta extends far beyond the realm of the physical, shaping the landscape of the mind and emotions with its fierce intensity and drive. Pitta types possess a sharp intellect and a keen analytical mind, with a natural talent for problem-solving and critical thinking. They are driven by a strong sense of purpose and are not afraid to pursue their goals with unwavering determination and focus. Yet, the same qualities that make Pitta types so dynamic and ambitious can also leave them susceptible to imbalances when in excess. In times of stress or frustration, Pitta individuals may experience feelings of anger, irritability, or impatience, as their fiery temperament flares up in response to perceived obstacles or challenges.

Balancing Pitta

In Ayurveda, maintaining balance within the Pitta dosha is seen as crucial for supporting overall health and well-being. This may involve incorporating cooling and soothing practices into daily life, such as engaging in calming activities like meditation or spending time in nature, and prioritizing cooling, hydrating foods in the diet. By honoring the unique qualities of Pitta and embracing practices that promote balance and harmony, individuals can harness the transformative power of this ancient wisdom, leading to a life filled with vitality, clarity, and fulfillment.

As we journey through the intricate landscape of Ayurvedic wisdom, the dosha of Pitta emerges as a fiery force of energy and transformation, guiding us towards greater understanding and self-awareness. By cultivating an awareness of our individual Pitta constitution and embracing practices that foster balance and harmony, we can unlock the full potential of this ancient wisdom, leading to a life filled with vitality, clarity, and fulfillment.

Kapha

Understanding Kapha

In the profound philosophy of Ayurveda, the dosha known as Kapha emerges as a stabilizing force of nourishment, endurance, and compassion. Comprised of the elemental energies of earth and water, Kapha governs the subtle rhythms of structure, cohesion, and stability within the human body and mind, shaping our experiences of strength, resilience, and connection with the world.

The Essence of Kapha

Kapha, with its grounding presence, serves as the foundation upon which the body and mind find their stability and equilibrium. Like the solid earth beneath our feet and the nourishing waters that flow through the land, Kapha provides us with a sense of rootedness, strength, and endurance, grounding us in the depths of our being. Individuals with a predominant Kapha constitution are often described as calm, compassionate, and nurturing, possessing a natural inclination towards caregiving and support.

Physical Characteristics

Physically, Kapha manifests itself through a unique interplay of qualities that reflect its elemental composition. Kapha types typically exhibit a sturdy, well-built physique, with broad shoulders and a solid, robust frame that exudes a sense of stability and strength. Their features are often characterized by soft, rounded contours and smooth, supple skin that radiates a sense of health and vitality. Yet, beneath this surface, Kapha individuals may also experience tendencies towards heaviness and stagnation, with a propensity for sluggish metabolism and weight gain.

Mental and Emotional Traits

The influence of Kapha extends far beyond the realm of the physical, shaping the landscape of the mind and emotions with its nurturing presence and emotional resilience. Kapha types possess a gentle, compassionate nature and are known for their steadfast loyalty and unwavering support for others. They approach life with a sense of calmness and contentment, finding joy and fulfillment in the simple pleasures of everyday living. Yet, the same qualities that make Kapha types so nurturing and empathetic can also leave them susceptible to imbalances when in excess. In times of stagnation or lethargy, Kapha individuals may experience feelings of attachment, inertia, or complacency, as their natural inclination towards stability tips into stagnation.

Balancing Kapha

In Ayurveda, maintaining balance within the Kapha dosha is seen as crucial for supporting overall health and well-being. This may involve incorporating invigorating and stimulating practices into daily life, such as engaging in regular exercise or practicing pranayama (breathwork), and prioritizing light, warming foods in the diet. By honoring the unique qualities of Kapha and embracing practices that promote balance and harmony, individuals can harness the transformative power of this ancient wisdom, leading to a life filled with vitality, resilience, and fulfillment.

As we journey through the intricate landscape of Ayurvedic wisdom, the dosha of Kapha emerges as a stabilizing force of nourishment and endurance, guiding us towards greater understanding and self-awareness. By cultivating an awareness of our individual Kapha constitution and embracing practices that foster balance and harmony, we can unlock the full potential of this ancient wisdom, leading to a life filled with vitality, resilience, and fulfillment.

Identifying Your Dominant Dosha

In the vast expanse of Ayurvedic wisdom, understanding your dominant dosha is akin to unlocking the blueprint of your individual constitution and well-being. Rooted in the elemental energies of nature, each dosha—Vata, Pitta, and Kapha—bestows upon us a unique combination of physical, mental, and emotional traits that shape our experiences of health and vitality. By gaining insight into your dominant dosha, you embark on a journey of self-discovery and empowerment, aligning yourself with the rhythms of nature and harnessing the transformative power of Ayurveda in your daily life.

The Three Doshas: Vata, Pitta, and Kapha

Before delving into the intricacies of identifying your dominant dosha, it's essential to gain a basic understanding of the three doshas and their respective qualities:

- **Vata**: Governed by the elements of air and ether, Vata embodies the qualities of movement, creativity, and change.
- **Pitta**: Rooted in the elements of fire and water, Pitta represents the forces of transformation, intensity, and intelligence.
- **Kapha**: Formed by the elements of earth and water, Kapha manifests as the energies of stability, nourishment, and endurance.

Self-Assessment: Recognizing Dosha Characteristics

Identifying your dominant dosha begins with self-awareness and observation. Take a moment to reflect on your physical, mental, and emotional traits, noting any patterns or tendencies that align with the qualities of Vata, Pitta, or Kapha:

- **Physical Characteristics**: Consider your body type, skin texture, hair quality, and other physical attributes. Are you slender and light like Vata, medium-built and intense like Pitta, or sturdy and grounded like Kapha?
- **Mental and Emotional Traits**: Reflect on your thought patterns, emotional responses, and behavioral tendencies. Are you creative and imaginative like Vata, driven and ambitious like Pitta, or nurturing and empathetic like Kapha?

Dosha Questionnaires and Assessments

For a more structured approach to identifying your dominant dosha, consider utilizing dosha questionnaires and assessments available in Ayurvedic literature or online resources. These tools typically consist of a series of questions designed to evaluate your physical, mental, and emotional characteristics and determine your doshic constitution.

Seeking Guidance from an Ayurvedic Practitioner

For a personalized and comprehensive assessment of your doshic constitution, consider consulting with an experienced Ayurvedic practitioner. Through pulse diagnosis, tongue examination, and detailed questioning, an Ayurvedic practitioner can provide insights into your unique constitution and offer guidance on lifestyle modifications, dietary recommendations, and holistic practices tailored to support your overall well-being.

Embracing Your Dosha and Living in Harmony

Whether you identify as predominantly Vata, Pitta, or Kapha, embracing your doshic constitution is an invitation to live in harmony with the natural rhythms of your body, mind, and spirit. By incorporating Ayurvedic principles into your daily life—such as following a dosha-balancing diet, practicing mindfulness and self-care, and cultivating a deep connection with nature—you can unlock the full potential of your dosha and embark on a journey of holistic wellness and vitality.

As you embark on the journey of identifying your dominant dosha, remember that Ayurveda is a dynamic and ever-evolving science that honors the uniqueness of each individual. Embrace the process with curiosity and openness, knowing that self-discovery is a lifelong journey filled with growth, insight, and transformation. By aligning yourself with the wisdom of Ayurveda and embracing the qualities of your dominant dosha, you pave the way for a life filled with balance, vitality, and radiant well-being.

Balancing Doshas in Daily Life

In the tapestry of Ayurveda, the art of balancing the doshas is a cornerstone of holistic wellness and vitality. Rooted in the elemental energies of nature, each dosha—Vata, Pitta, and Kapha—bestows upon us a unique constitution that shapes our physical, mental, and emotional well-being. By cultivating awareness and incorporating Ayurvedic principles into our daily lives, we can harmonize the doshas and unlock the transformative power of ancient wisdom in our modern existence.

Embracing Dosha-Balancing Practices

Balancing the doshas begins with embracing practices that honor the unique qualities and tendencies of each dosha. Whether you identify as predominantly Vata, Pitta, or Kapha, incorporating dosha-balancing practices into your daily routine can help restore harmony and equilibrium within the body and mind.

- **Vata-Balancing Practices**: For individuals with a dominant Vata constitution, grounding and nourishing practices are key. Establishing a regular routine, engaging in gentle exercise like yoga or walking in nature, and prioritizing warm, cooked foods can help pacify excess Vata and promote stability and calmness.
- **Pitta-Balancing Practices**: If Pitta predominates in your constitution, focus on cooling and soothing practices to balance the fiery energy of Pitta. Incorporating mindfulness techniques such as meditation or deep breathing, avoiding spicy and acidic foods, and spending time in nature can help alleviate Pitta imbalances and promote a sense of balance and clarity.
- **Kapha-Balancing Practices**: For those with a dominant Kapha constitution, invigorating and stimulating practices are essential. Engage in regular exercise that gets your blood flowing, incorporate warming spices like ginger and cinnamon into your diet, and cultivate a sense of purpose and motivation to counteract feelings of lethargy and stagnation.

Mindful Eating for Dosha Balance

Diet plays a crucial role in balancing the doshas and supporting overall well-being. By incorporating dosha-balancing foods into your meals and being mindful of your eating habits, you can nourish your body and promote harmony within the doshas.

- **Vata-Pacifying Foods**: Opt for warm, cooked foods that are grounding and nourishing, such as grains like rice and oats, root vegetables like sweet potatoes and carrots, and warming spices like ginger and cinnamon.
- **Pitta-Pacifying Foods**: Choose cooling and hydrating foods that soothe the fiery nature of Pitta, such as leafy greens, sweet fruits like melons and berries, and cooling herbs like mint and cilantro.
- **Kapha-Pacifying Foods**: Focus on light and stimulating foods that counteract the heaviness of Kapha, such as legumes, leafy greens, spicy foods like chili peppers, and pungent herbs like garlic and mustard.

Holistic Self-Care Practices

In addition to diet and lifestyle modifications, incorporating holistic self-care practices can further support dosha balance and overall well-being. Explore Ayurvedic rituals such as self-massage with warm oils (Abhyanga), tongue scraping, and oil pulling to nourish and detoxify the body, mind, and senses.

Cultivating Awareness and Adaptability

Ultimately, balancing the doshas is a dynamic and ongoing process that requires awareness, adaptability, and a willingness to listen to the needs of your body and mind. By cultivating mindfulness and embracing the wisdom of Ayurveda, you can navigate life's ebbs and flows with grace and resilience, fostering a deep sense of vitality and well-being in every moment.

As you integrate dosha-balancing practices into your daily life, remember that Ayurveda is not a one-size-fits-all approach but rather a personalized journey of self-discovery and empowerment. Embrace the uniqueness of your doshic constitution and honor the wisdom of your body and mind as you embark on this transformative path towards holistic wellness and radiant living.

Part 2: Daily Ayurvedic Practices

1. Morning Routines for Wellness

Dinacharya: The Ayurvedic Daily Routine

In Ayurveda, the daily routine, or Dinacharya, is considered a cornerstone of good health and wellness. This ancient practice involves aligning one's daily activities with the natural cycles of the day and night. According to Ayurvedic wisdom, following a consistent daily routine helps maintain balance among the doshas—Vata, Pitta, and Kapha—thereby promoting overall well-being and preventing disease. A well-structured morning routine sets the tone for the rest of the day, grounding and energizing the body and mind.

The Ayurvedic morning begins before sunrise, in a period known as Brahma Muhurta. This time, approximately 96 minutes before sunrise, is considered the most auspicious for spiritual practices and self-reflection. The environment is calm, and the mind is naturally still, making it an ideal time for meditation, prayer, or quiet contemplation. Rising during this period helps to harmonize the body's internal rhythms with the natural world, fostering a sense of peace and clarity.

Upon waking, the first step in the Ayurvedic morning routine is to express gratitude. This simple act of thankfulness for the new day sets a positive and mindful tone, fostering a sense of peace and contentment. Following this, it is recommended to drink a glass of warm water, which helps to stimulate the digestive system, flush out toxins, and rehydrate the body after a night's rest.

Next, Ayurvedic tradition emphasizes oral hygiene practices such as tongue scraping and oil pulling. Tongue scraping involves using a special tool to gently scrape the surface of the tongue, removing accumulated toxins, or ama, that can build up overnight. This not only freshens the breath but also enhances the sense of taste and stimulates the digestive system. Oil pulling, another key practice, involves swishing a tablespoon of oil, typically sesame or coconut oil, in the mouth for about 15-20 minutes. This practice is believed to draw out toxins, improve oral health, and strengthen the teeth and gums.

Following oral hygiene, the next step is to cleanse the nasal passages using a neti pot, a practice known as Jala Neti. This involves pouring warm saline water through one nostril and letting it flow out the other, clearing the nasal passages of mucus and impurities. Jala Neti helps to improve breathing, enhance mental clarity, and prevent sinus infections.

Abhyanga, or self-massage with warm oil, is a deeply nourishing and grounding practice recommended in the Ayurvedic morning routine. The type of oil used can be tailored to one's dosha: sesame oil for Vata, coconut oil for Pitta, and mustard or sunflower oil for Kapha. Gently massaging the oil into the skin using circular motions on the joints and long strokes on the limbs helps to improve circulation, nourish the skin, calm the nervous system, and promote lymphatic drainage. After the massage, it is beneficial to allow the oil to soak in for a few minutes before taking a warm shower or bath to cleanse the body and remove the excess oil.

Exercise is another vital component of the Ayurvedic morning routine. The type and intensity of exercise should be suited to one's constitution. Vata types benefit from gentle, grounding exercises like yoga, tai chi, or walking. Pitta types can engage in moderate activities that do not overheat the body, such as swimming, cycling, or brisk walking. Kapha types often require more vigorous exercise to stimulate their naturally slower metabolism, including running, aerobics, or intense yoga. Regular physical activity helps to maintain balance in the doshas, improve circulation, enhance digestion, and boost overall energy levels.

After exercise, it is recommended to practice pranayama, or breath control exercises, to harmonize the flow of energy within the body. Techniques such as Nadi Shodhana (alternate nostril breathing) help to balance the doshas, calm the mind, and increase mental clarity. Kapalabhati (skull shining breath) invigorates and detoxifies, making it particularly beneficial for Kapha types.

Following pranayama, spending a few minutes in meditation can greatly enhance mental clarity and emotional resilience. Meditation helps to quiet the mind, reduce stress, and cultivate a state of inner peace and awareness. This practice can be as simple as focusing on the breath, repeating a mantra, or observing the thoughts without attachment.

The Ayurvedic morning routine culminates with a nourishing breakfast tailored to one's dosha. Vata types benefit from warm, grounding foods such as oatmeal with ghee and warming spices like cinnamon and cardamom. Pitta types should opt for cooling and soothing foods like fresh fruits, soaked almonds, and light grains. Kapha types need light and energizing foods, such as spiced herbal teas and quinoa porridge, to stimulate their metabolism.

In summary, the Ayurvedic morning routine, or Dinacharya, is a comprehensive practice designed to align the body and mind with the natural rhythms of the day. By incorporating practices such as gratitude, hydration, oral hygiene, nasal cleansing, self-massage, exercise, pranayama, meditation, and a dosha-specific breakfast, individuals can cultivate a balanced and harmonious start to their day. These practices not only promote physical health but also enhance mental clarity and emotional well-being, laying a strong foundation for overall wellness. Embracing Dinacharya is a powerful way to harness the ancient wisdom of Ayurveda to support a vibrant, balanced, and fulfilling life.

Morning Practices: Tongue Scraping, Oil Pulling, and Abhyanga (Self-Massage)

As the first rays of sunlight filter through the curtains, heralding the dawn of a new day, we are presented with a sacred opportunity to cultivate wellness and vitality through the ancient practices of Ayurveda. In the stillness of the early morning, before the hustle and bustle of daily life ensues, lies a precious moment to connect with ourselves and set the tone for the day ahead. This chapter delves into the transformative power of morning rituals, focusing on three key practices: Tongue Scraping, Oil Pulling, and Abhyanga (Self-Massage).

Awakening the Senses: Tongue Scraping

In the gentle embrace of dawn, as we awaken from our slumber, our senses come alive, eager to greet the day. Among the myriad practices that form the cornerstone of Ayurvedic daily routines, tongue scraping stands out as a simple yet profoundly effective ritual for promoting oral and overall health.

Tongue scraping, or Jihwa Prakshalana, is a centuries-old Ayurvedic practice that involves gently removing the accumulated toxins and bacteria from the surface of the tongue. This simple act not only cleanses the oral cavity but also stimulates the digestive organs, enhances taste perception, and promotes fresh breath.

Using a tongue scraper made of copper, silver, or stainless steel, practitioners gently scrape the tongue from back to front, removing the thin film of debris that accumulates overnight. As the toxins are expelled, a sense of clarity and freshness pervades the senses, preparing the body and mind for the day ahead.

Nourishing the Body: Oil Pulling

Following the cleansing ritual of tongue scraping, Ayurvedic wisdom invites us to nourish and purify the body from within through the practice of oil pulling, or Gandusha. Originating from the ancient text of Charaka Samhita, oil pulling involves swishing a tablespoon of warm, organic oil (such as sesame, coconut, or sunflower oil) in the mouth for 10 to 20 minutes, before spitting it out.

Oil pulling serves as a natural detoxifier, drawing out impurities and harmful bacteria from the oral cavity, while also moisturizing the gums and promoting oral hygiene. Beyond its benefits for dental health, oil pulling is believed to stimulate the lymphatic system, boost the immune system, and promote overall well-being.

As the oil glides through the mouth, coating every surface with its nourishing embrace, practitioners experience a sense of renewal and vitality, aligning themselves with the natural rhythms of the body and the universe.

Cultivating Self-Care: Abhyanga (Self-Massage)

As the final act of our morning ritual unfolds, we are invited to indulge in the luxurious practice of Abhyanga, or self-massage—an integral aspect of Ayurvedic self-care and wellness. Derived from the Sanskrit words 'Abhi' (meaning 'towards') and 'Anga' (meaning 'limb'), Abhyanga involves massaging warm, herb-infused oils into the skin, from head to toe, in a rhythmic and intentional manner.

Abhyanga not only nourishes the skin and soothes the muscles but also calms the nervous system, balances the doshas (Ayurvedic body types), and promotes emotional well-being. By incorporating this self-care ritual into our morning routine, we cultivate a deeper sense of connection with ourselves and honor the body as a sacred vessel of healing and transformation.

As the fragrant oils envelop our senses, penetrating deep into the layers of our being, we are reminded of the profound wisdom inherent in the practice of Ayurveda. With each stroke of our hands, we infuse ourselves with love and intention, embracing the journey of self-discovery and holistic wellness.

In the tapestry of daily life, the morning rituals of Ayurveda serve as anchors of stability and sources of inspiration, guiding us on a journey of self-care and self-discovery. Through the practices of tongue scraping, oil pulling, and Abhyanga, we awaken to the innate wisdom of our bodies and align ourselves with the rhythms of nature.

As we embark on this journey of holistic wellness, may we approach each morning with reverence and gratitude, honoring the ancient teachings of Ayurveda and embracing the transformative power of daily rituals. In doing so, we pave the way for a life filled with vitality, balance, and radiant well-being.

Ayurvedic Breakfasts

In the tranquil moments of early morning, before the world awakens in a flurry of activity, lies an opportune time to cultivate wellness and set the tone for the day ahead. Ayurveda, the ancient science of life, offers a rich tapestry of practices designed to nurture body, mind, and spirit during this sacred time. Among these practices, the choices we make for breakfast play a pivotal role in sustaining our vitality and aligning us with the rhythms of nature.

The Ayurvedic Approach to Breakfast

In Ayurveda, breakfast is considered the most important meal of the day, providing the nourishment and sustenance needed to fuel our bodies and minds as we embark on our daily journey. Unlike the hurried and often haphazard breakfasts of modern living, Ayurvedic breakfasts are crafted with intention, balancing the doshas (Ayurvedic body types) and harmonizing the elements within us.

Nourishing the Doshas: Tailoring Breakfast to Your Constitution

Central to the Ayurvedic approach to breakfast is the recognition that each individual possesses a unique constitution, or Prakriti, composed of varying proportions of the three doshas: Vata, Pitta, and Kapha. By understanding our constitution and the prevailing doshic influences of the current season, we can tailor our breakfast choices to support balance and well-being.

For Vata individuals, who tend to be creative and energetic yet prone to anxiety and irregular digestion, a grounding and nourishing breakfast is key. Warm, cooked grains such as oatmeal or rice porridge, topped with ghee (clarified butter), cinnamon, and nuts, provide the stability and comfort needed to start the day on a centered note.

Pitta types, characterized by their intensity, intelligence, and fiery nature, benefit from cooling and soothing breakfast options that help to pacify excess heat and acidity. A refreshing fruit salad with coconut flakes, a dollop of yogurt, and a sprinkle of cardamom offers a light yet satisfying start to the day, promoting balance and clarity of mind.

For Kapha individuals, who possess strength and endurance yet may struggle with sluggish digestion and lethargy, a stimulating and invigorating breakfast is ideal. A warm bowl of spiced quinoa or barley porridge, infused with ginger, turmeric, and a touch of honey, awakens the senses and enlivens the body, setting the stage for productivity and vitality.

Embracing Seasonal Eating: The Wisdom of Nature

In addition to honoring our individual constitutions, Ayurveda emphasizes the importance of eating seasonally, aligning our diets with the natural rhythms of the earth. Just as the seasons transition and evolve, so too should our breakfast choices, reflecting the qualities and energies prevalent in nature at any given time.

During the abundant growth of spring and summer, when the earth is fertile and vibrant, we are drawn to light and refreshing breakfasts that cool and nourish the body. Fresh fruits, leafy greens, and smoothies bursting with vitality provide the perfect complement to the warmth and expansiveness of these seasons, promoting detoxification and rejuvenation.

As the seasons shift towards autumn and winter, and the energies of the earth begin to contract and withdraw, our breakfast choices naturally gravitate towards warmer, heartier options that offer comfort and sustenance. Root vegetables, hearty soups, and warm grain bowls infused with aromatic spices provide the grounding nourishment needed to navigate the cooler months with resilience and vitality.

In the rhythm of daily life, the choices we make for breakfast serve as a reflection of our commitment to holistic well-being and alignment with the wisdom of Ayurveda. By honoring our individual constitutions, embracing seasonal eating, and approaching each meal with mindfulness and intention, we nourish not only our bodies but also our souls, cultivating a deep sense of vitality and harmony that permeates every aspect of our lives.

As we embark on this journey of conscious living, may we savor each bite with gratitude and reverence, honoring the ancient wisdom of Ayurveda and embracing the transformative power of daily rituals. In doing so, we nourish not only our bodies but also our spirits, forging a path towards radiant health, balance, and fulfillment.

2. Ayurvedic Nutrition

The Six Tastes in Ayurveda

Exploring the Six Tastes

In the realm of Ayurveda, nutrition is not merely about fueling the body but also about nourishing the soul and fostering balance within the doshas. Central to Ayurvedic nutrition is the concept of the six tastes, each with its unique qualities and effects on the body and mind. By incorporating a variety of tastes into our meals, we can support optimal digestion, promote dosha balance, and cultivate overall well-being.

Understanding the Six Tastes

The six tastes—sweet, sour, salty, bitter, pungent, and astringent—are derived from the five elements of nature and play a crucial role in Ayurvedic nutrition. Each taste carries specific qualities and has a distinct impact on the doshas, influencing our physical health, mental clarity, and emotional balance.

1. **Sweet (Madhura)**: The sweet taste is characterized by its grounding and nourishing qualities. Foods with a sweet taste provide stability and energy, promote tissue growth, and pacify Vata and Pitta doshas. Examples include grains like rice and wheat, root vegetables like sweet potatoes and carrots, and sweet fruits like bananas and dates.
2. **Sour (Amla)**: The sour taste is acidic and stimulating, promoting digestion and metabolic function. Foods with a sour taste enhance appetite, aid in digestion, and stimulate the senses. Sour taste also aggravates Pitta but can balance Vata and Kapha in moderation. Examples include citrus fruits like lemons and oranges, yogurt, vinegar, and fermented foods.
3. **Salty (Lavana)**: The salty taste is heating and hydrating, supporting electrolyte balance and fluid regulation in the body. Foods with a salty taste stimulate digestion, promote hydration, and can alleviate Vata and enhance Pitta, but can aggravate

Kapha in excess. Examples include sea salt, seaweed, miso, and olives.
4. **Bitter (Tikta)**: The bitter taste is cooling and detoxifying, helping to purify the blood and cleanse the body of toxins. Foods with a bitter taste promote detoxification, reduce inflammation, and balance Pitta and Kapha, but can aggravate Vata in excess. Examples include leafy greens like kale and spinach, bitter melon, turmeric, and dandelion greens.
5. **Pungent (Katu)**: The pungent taste is heating and stimulating, promoting circulation and metabolism. Foods with a pungent taste stimulate digestion, improve circulation, and balance Kapha and Vata, but can aggravate Pitta in excess. Examples include spices like chili peppers, ginger, garlic, and black pepper.
6. **Astringent (Kashaya)**: The astringent taste is drying and tonifying, helping to absorb excess moisture and promote tissue firmness. Foods with an astringent taste promote healing, reduce inflammation, and balance Pitta and Kapha, but can aggravate Vata in excess. Examples include legumes like lentils and beans, green tea, pomegranates, and cranberries.

Balancing the Six Tastes

In Ayurvedic nutrition, the key to dosha balance lies in incorporating all six tastes into our meals in appropriate proportions. By embracing a variety of tastes, we can support optimal digestion, promote dosha balance, and cultivate overall well-being. A well-balanced meal ideally includes all six tastes, with an emphasis on tastes that balance our individual doshic constitution.

For example, a meal for a Pitta-dominant individual might include cooling and hydrating foods with sweet, bitter, and astringent tastes to pacify Pitta's fiery nature. Conversely, a meal for a Vata-dominant individual might incorporate grounding and nourishing foods with sweet, sour, and salty tastes to stabilize Vata's airy qualities.

Mindful Eating for Dosha Balance

In addition to embracing the six tastes, Ayurvedic nutrition emphasizes the importance of mindful eating practices to support optimal digestion and dosha balance. By eating slowly, savoring each bite, and paying attention to the qualities of the food, we can enhance our digestive fire (Agni) and promote the assimilation of nutrients.

As we explore the six tastes in Ayurvedic nutrition, we uncover a wealth of wisdom that empowers us to nourish our bodies, minds, and spirits in harmony with the rhythms of nature. By embracing a variety of tastes and adopting mindful eating practices, we can support optimal digestion, promote dosha balance, and cultivate overall well-being in our daily lives. Through the transformative power of Ayurvedic nutrition, we embark on a journey of holistic wellness and radiant living, honoring the ancient wisdom that guides us towards health, harmony, and vitality.

Eating for Your Dosha

Ayurvedic Nutrition: Eating for Your Dosha

In the rich tapestry of Ayurveda, nutrition is not just about satisfying hunger; it is a sacred practice that nourishes the body, mind, and spirit, fostering balance and harmony within. Central to Ayurvedic nutrition is the recognition that each individual possesses a unique constitution, or dosha, which influences their dietary needs, preferences, and responses to food. By understanding and honoring our doshic constitution, we can cultivate optimal health and vitality through mindful eating practices that support dosha balance and holistic well-being.

Embracing Individuality: The Three Doshas

Before delving into eating for your dosha, it's essential to gain a basic understanding of the three doshas—Vata, Pitta, and Kapha—and their respective qualities:

- **Vata**: Governed by the elements of air and ether, Vata is characterized by qualities of movement, creativity, and change.
- **Pitta**: Rooted in the elements of fire and water, Pitta embodies the forces of transformation, intensity, and intelligence.
- **Kapha**: Formed by the elements of earth and water, Kapha manifests as the energies of stability, nourishment, and endurance.

Eating for Your Dosha: A Personalized Approach

Eating for your dosha involves aligning your diet with the unique qualities and tendencies of your dominant dosha while also considering any imbalances that may be present. By incorporating foods that balance and pacify your dominant dosha, you can support optimal digestion, promote dosha harmony, and cultivate overall well-being.

- **Vata-Pacifying Diet**: For individuals with a predominant Vata constitution, focus on grounding and nourishing foods that provide stability and warmth. Emphasize cooked grains like rice and oats, root vegetables like sweet potatoes and carrots, and warm, moist

foods like soups and stews. Avoid cold, dry, and raw foods, which can exacerbate Vata imbalances.
- **Pitta-Pacifying Diet**: If Pitta predominates in your constitution, opt for cooling and soothing foods that balance Pitta's fiery nature. Incorporate sweet, bitter, and astringent tastes into your meals, with an emphasis on fresh fruits and vegetables, whole grains like quinoa and barley, and cooling herbs and spices like mint and coriander. Limit spicy, acidic, and fried foods, which can aggravate Pitta imbalances.
- **Kapha-Pacifying Diet**: For those with a dominant Kapha constitution, focus on light and stimulating foods that counteract Kapha's heavy qualities. Embrace a diet rich in pungent, bitter, and astringent tastes, with an emphasis on leafy greens, legumes, light grains like millet and buckwheat, and warming spices like ginger and black pepper. Minimize heavy, oily, and sweet foods, which can exacerbate Kapha imbalances.

Mindful Eating Practices

In addition to aligning your diet with your doshic constitution, practicing mindful eating can further support dosha balance and overall well-being. Mindful eating involves cultivating awareness and presence during meals, savoring each bite, and listening to your body's hunger and fullness cues. By slowing down and tuning into the sensory experience of eating, you can enhance digestion, promote nutrient absorption, and foster a deeper connection with your food and your body.

Cultivating Balance and Harmony

As you embark on the journey of eating for your dosha, remember that Ayurveda is a dynamic and personalized science that honors the uniqueness of each individual. Embrace experimentation and self-discovery as you explore the foods and flavors that resonate with your doshic constitution, and listen to the wisdom of your body as you nourish yourself with love and intention.

By embracing the principles of Ayurvedic nutrition and eating for your dosha, you embark on a journey of self-discovery and empowerment that fosters balance, harmony, and vitality in every aspect of your being. Through mindful eating practices that honor your doshic constitution and support dosha balance, you cultivate a deeper connection with yourself and the world around you, leading to a life filled with health, happiness, and radiant well-being.

Seasonal Eating

In the timeless tradition of Ayurveda, the concept of seasonal eating is deeply ingrained, recognizing the dynamic interplay between the changing seasons and our dietary needs. By aligning our diet with the rhythms of nature, we can support optimal health and well-being, promote dosha balance, and cultivate a deeper connection with the natural world. In this chapter, we explore the principles of seasonal eating in Ayurveda and how they can guide us towards a more nourishing and harmonious relationship with food.

Honoring Nature's Rhythms

Ayurveda teaches us that the qualities of the natural world are constantly in flux, with each season bringing its unique combination of elements and energies. By attuning our diet to the seasonal changes around us, we can adapt to these shifting rhythms and support our body's natural ability to maintain balance and vitality.

- **Spring**: As nature awakens from its winter slumber, the qualities of Kapha dosha predominate, bringing moisture, heaviness, and stability. During the spring season, focus on lightening up your diet with cleansing and detoxifying foods, such as bitter greens, sprouts, and pungent spices, to balance Kapha's heavy qualities and support the body's natural cleansing processes.
- **Summer**: With the heat of summer comes the intensity of Pitta dosha, characterized by heat, intensity, and transformation. During the summer months, opt for cooling and hydrating foods like fresh fruits and vegetables, coconut water, and mint-infused drinks to pacify Pitta's fiery nature and maintain balance in the body.
- **Autumn**: As the leaves begin to fall and the air becomes crisp, the qualities of Vata dosha become more prominent, bringing dryness, mobility, and change. During the autumn season, focus on grounding and nourishing foods like root vegetables, hearty grains, and warming spices to counteract Vata's airy qualities and support stability and grounding.

- **Winter**: With the arrival of winter, the qualities of Kapha dosha return, bringing cold, dampness, and heaviness. During the winter months, embrace warming and comforting foods like soups, stews, and cooked grains to pacify Kapha's cold and heavy qualities and promote warmth and nourishment in the body.

Adapting to Seasonal Changes

In addition to adjusting our diet to the changing seasons, Ayurveda teaches us to listen to the cues of our body and adapt our eating habits accordingly. Pay attention to your body's cravings, energy levels, and digestive capacity, and make adjustments to your diet as needed to support balance and well-being.

- **Spring**: Incorporate cleansing and detoxifying foods like bitter greens, dandelion greens, and cruciferous vegetables into your diet to support the body's natural detoxification processes and lighten the load on the digestive system.
- **Summer**: Embrace cooling and hydrating foods like cucumber, watermelon, and coconut water to stay hydrated and cool during the hot summer months. Limit spicy and heavy foods that can aggravate Pitta and contribute to heat-related imbalances.
- **Autumn**: Focus on grounding and nourishing foods like root vegetables, squash, and hearty grains to support stability and grounding during the season of change. Incorporate warming spices like cinnamon, ginger, and nutmeg to promote digestion and maintain warmth in the body.
- **Winter**: Indulge in warming and comforting foods like soups, stews, and casseroles to stay cozy and nourished during the cold winter months. Incorporate nourishing fats like ghee and coconut oil to support immunity and provide insulation against the cold.

Cultivating Awareness and Connection

By embracing the principles of seasonal eating, we not only support our physical health but also cultivate a deeper connection with the natural world and the cycles of life. As we tune into the rhythms of nature and honor the wisdom of our body's innate intelligence, we embark on a journey of holistic wellness and radiant living, nourished by the bountiful gifts of the earth.

Seasonal eating is a cornerstone of Ayurvedic nutrition, guiding us towards a more nourishing and harmonious relationship with food and the natural world. By aligning our diet with the changing seasons and adapting to the rhythms of nature, we can support optimal health and vitality, promote dosha balance, and cultivate a deeper sense of connection and well-being in every aspect of our lives. Through the transformative power of seasonal eating, we honor the ancient wisdom of Ayurveda and embark on a journey of holistic wellness and radiant living.

3. Midday Practices for Energy

Ayurvedic Lunch Tips

As the midday sun reaches its zenith, our bodies crave nourishment and rejuvenation to sustain us through the remainder of the day. In Ayurveda, the midday meal holds a special significance as an opportunity to replenish our energy reserves, support digestion, and balance the doshas. In this chapter, we explore Ayurvedic lunch tips and practices to promote vitality, clarity, and well-being during the busiest hours of the day.

The Importance of the Midday Meal

In Ayurveda, the midday meal is considered the most substantial and nourishing meal of the day, providing the body with essential nutrients and energy to fuel physical and mental activities. As the digestive fire (Agni) reaches its peak during the middle of the day, our bodies are primed to efficiently digest and assimilate food, making this an ideal time to enjoy a hearty and satisfying meal.

Balancing the Doshas with Lunch

When planning your midday meal, it's essential to consider your doshic constitution and any imbalances that may be present. By incorporating foods and flavors that support dosha balance, you can promote optimal digestion, enhance energy levels, and cultivate a sense of well-being.

- **Vata-Pacifying Lunch**: For individuals with a predominant Vata constitution, opt for warm, nourishing foods that provide stability and grounding. Incorporate cooked grains like rice or quinoa, cooked vegetables, and warming spices like ginger and cumin to pacify Vata's airy qualities and support digestion.
- **Pitta-Pacifying Lunch**: If Pitta predominates in your constitution, focus on cooling and hydrating foods that soothe Pitta's fiery nature. Include plenty of fresh fruits and vegetables, whole grains like barley or couscous, and cooling herbs like cilantro and mint to pacify Pitta and maintain balance in the body.

- **Kapha-Pacifying Lunch**: For those with a dominant Kapha constitution, embrace light and stimulating foods that counteract Kapha's heavy qualities. Incorporate plenty of leafy greens, legumes, and pungent spices like ginger and black pepper to stimulate digestion and promote vitality.

Mindful Eating Practices

In addition to selecting dosha-balancing foods, practicing mindful eating during the midday meal can further support digestion, energy levels, and overall well-being. Take time to savor each bite, chew your food thoroughly, and eat in a calm and relaxed environment to enhance digestion and promote satiety.

Incorporating Ayurvedic Lunch Tips

When preparing and enjoying your midday meal, consider incorporating the following Ayurvedic lunch tips to optimize energy and vitality:

- **Eat at Regular Intervals**: Aim to eat your midday meal at the same time each day to support healthy digestion and maintain stable energy levels.
- **Include a Variety of Flavors**: Embrace the six tastes—sweet, sour, salty, bitter, pungent, and astringent—in your midday meal to ensure balance and satisfaction.
- **Stay Hydrated**: Drink warm water or herbal teas with your meal to aid digestion and prevent dehydration.
- **Eat Mindfully**: Take time to appreciate the flavors, textures, and aromas of your food, and listen to your body's hunger and fullness cues to avoid overeating.
- **Enjoy a Restful Afternoon**: After your midday meal, take a short break to rest and rejuvenate, allowing your body to digest and assimilate food before returning to your daily activities.

The midday meal is a sacred opportunity to nourish and replenish our bodies, supporting energy, vitality, and well-being during the busiest hours of the day. By incorporating Ayurvedic lunch tips and practices into our daily routine, we can honor the wisdom of our body's innate intelligence and cultivate a deeper connection with the nourishing gifts of food and nature. Through the transformative power of mindful eating and dosha-balancing nutrition, we embark on a journey of holistic wellness and radiant living, guided by the ancient wisdom of Ayurveda.

Importance of Agni (Digestive Fire)

In the bustling rhythm of modern life, the midday hours offer a brief respite—a moment to pause, nourish ourselves, and replenish our energy reserves for the tasks that lie ahead. At the heart of this nourishment lies Agni, the transformative power of digestion that converts food into energy, vitality, and life force. In this chapter, we delve into the significance of Agni and explore midday practices that support its optimal function, promoting energy, clarity, and well-being.

Understanding Agni: The Digestive Fire

In Ayurveda, Agni is revered as the cornerstone of health and vitality—a sacred fire that resides within the gastrointestinal tract and governs the process of digestion and metabolism. Like a flickering flame, Agni transforms the food we consume into nutrients that nourish our tissues, cells, and organs, providing the foundation for physical and mental well-being.

The Three Forms of Agni

Agni exists in three main forms within the body, each playing a distinct role in the digestive process:

1. **Jathara Agni (Gastric Fire)**: Located in the stomach, Jathara Agni initiates the process of digestion by breaking down food into smaller particles and preparing it for further digestion and absorption.
2. **Bhuta Agni (Tissue Fire)**: Bhuta Agni resides in the cells and tissues of the body, where it metabolizes nutrients and converts them into the building blocks of life, supporting growth, repair, and regeneration.
3. **Dhatu Agni (Metabolic Fire)**: Dhatu Agni governs the metabolic processes that occur within the tissues and organs,

regulating energy production, waste elimination, and cellular function.

Signs of Balanced Agni

When Agni is in a state of balance, it manifests as robust digestion, strong appetite, and regular elimination. Individuals with balanced Agni experience optimal energy levels, clear mental focus, and a sense of lightness and vitality after meals. They also enjoy strong immunity, efficient metabolism, and overall well-being.

Supporting Agni: Midday Practices for Energy

To support the optimal function of Agni and promote energy and vitality during the midday hours, consider incorporating the following practices into your daily routine:

- **Eat Mindfully**: Take time to eat your midday meal in a calm and relaxed environment, free from distractions. Chew your food thoroughly and savor each bite to enhance digestion and absorption of nutrients.
- **Choose Agni-Boosting Foods**: Opt for foods that kindle Agni and support digestive function, such as warming spices like ginger, cumin, and black pepper; cooked vegetables; whole grains; and nourishing soups and stews.
- **Stay Hydrated**: Drink warm water or herbal teas with your meal to support digestion and prevent dehydration. Avoid drinking excessive amounts of cold or iced beverages, as they can dampen Agni and impair digestion.
- **Engage in Gentle Movement**: Take a short walk or engage in gentle stretching exercises after your midday meal to stimulate digestion and promote circulation. Avoid vigorous exercise immediately after eating, as it can divert blood flow away from the digestive organs.
- **Cultivate Gratitude**: Before eating, take a moment to express gratitude for the nourishment provided by your food and the abundance of blessings in your life. Cultivating a mindset of gratitude can enhance the digestive process and promote a sense of well-being.

As we honor the transformative power of Agni and embrace midday practices that support its optimal function, we nourish not only our bodies but also our spirits, fostering energy, vitality, and well-being in every moment. By cultivating awareness and mindfulness around our eating habits and embracing the wisdom of Ayurveda, we tap into the innate intelligence of our body and align ourselves with the rhythms of nature, leading to a life filled with health, happiness, and radiant living.

Herbal Teas and Remedies

In the midst of a busy day, when energy wanes and concentration falters, a soothing cup of herbal tea can be a revitalizing elixir—a moment of nourishment and rejuvenation for body, mind, and spirit. Drawing upon the healing properties of medicinal herbs and spices, herbal teas offer a natural and gentle way to support energy levels, promote digestion, and enhance overall well-being. In this chapter, we explore the art of herbal teas and remedies as midday practices for sustained energy and vitality.

Harnessing the Healing Power of Herbs

For centuries, cultures around the world have revered medicinal herbs for their therapeutic properties and healing benefits. In Ayurveda, herbal remedies are prized for their ability to balance the doshas, support digestion, and promote vitality and longevity. By incorporating herbal teas into our midday routine, we can tap into the wisdom of nature and harness the healing power of plants to enhance energy levels and promote holistic well-being.

Ayurvedic Principles of Herbal Remedies

In Ayurveda, herbal remedies are prescribed based on an individual's unique constitution (Prakriti) and any imbalances that may be present. By selecting herbs and spices that align with the qualities and tendencies of the doshas, we can support optimal health and vitality in body and mind.

- **Vata-Balancing Herbs**: For individuals with a predominant Vata constitution, choose grounding and nourishing herbs like ashwagandha, shatavari, and licorice to promote stability, calmness, and resilience.

- **Pitta-Pacifying Herbs**: If Pitta predominates in your constitution, opt for cooling and soothing herbs like peppermint, coriander, and fennel to pacify Pitta's fiery nature and promote balance and harmony.
- **Kapha-Reducing Herbs**: For those with a dominant Kapha constitution, embrace invigorating and stimulating herbs like ginger, cinnamon, and clove to counteract Kapha's heavy qualities and promote energy and vitality.

Herbal Teas for Midday Energy

When selecting herbal teas for midday energy, consider the following options:

- **Ginger Tea**: Known for its warming and invigorating properties, ginger tea stimulates digestion, enhances circulation, and boosts energy levels. Simply steep fresh ginger slices in hot water for a revitalizing pick-me-up.
- **Tulsi (Holy Basil) Tea**: Revered as a sacred herb in Ayurveda, tulsi tea promotes mental clarity, reduces stress, and supports overall well-being. Enjoy a cup of tulsi tea to uplift the spirits and enhance focus and concentration.
- **Peppermint Tea**: Refreshing and cooling, peppermint tea aids digestion, relieves indigestion, and promotes mental alertness. Sip on a cup of peppermint tea to invigorate the senses and combat midday fatigue.
- **Cinnamon Tea**: Rich in antioxidants and warming spices, cinnamon tea enhances circulation, regulates blood sugar levels, and promotes vitality and warmth. Enjoy a comforting cup of cinnamon tea to boost energy and uplift the mood.

Making Herbal Teas: A Simple Guide

To prepare herbal teas, follow these simple steps:

1. **Choose Your Herbs**: Select your desired herbs and spices based on your doshic constitution and specific health goals.
2. **Steep**: Place the herbs in a teapot or infuser and pour hot water over them.

3. **Cover and Steep**: Cover the teapot and let the herbs steep for 5-10 minutes to allow the flavors and medicinal properties to infuse into the water.
4. **Strain and Serve**: Once steeped, strain the herbs from the tea and pour into a cup. Sweeten with honey or add a splash of lemon juice if desired.

As we embrace the healing power of herbal teas and remedies as midday practices for sustained energy and vitality, we honor the wisdom of nature and the innate intelligence of our body and mind. By incorporating Ayurvedic principles and selecting herbs and spices that support dosha balance, we can enhance our well-being and cultivate a deeper connection with the healing gifts of the earth. Through the transformative power of herbal teas, we embark on a journey of holistic wellness and radiant living, nourished by the bountiful abundance of nature's pharmacy.

4. Evening Routines for Rest:

Calming Practices Before Bed

As the sun sets and the day draws to a close, the evening hours offer a sacred opportunity for rest, renewal, and rejuvenation. In the ancient tradition of Ayurveda, the transition from day to night is a time to unwind, release tension, and prepare the body and mind for a restful night's sleep. In this chapter, we explore calming practices before bed and evening routines for rest that promote deep relaxation, tranquility, and inner peace.

The Importance of Evening Routines

In our fast-paced modern world, where stress and busyness often dominate our days, the evening hours provide a precious opportunity to slow down, reconnect with ourselves, and transition gracefully into a state of rest and relaxation. By establishing evening routines that honor the natural rhythms of our body and mind, we can create a sanctuary of peace and tranquility that supports deep, restorative sleep and overall well-being.

Calming Practices Before Bed

Incorporating calming practices before bed can help signal to the body and mind that it is time to unwind and prepare for sleep. Consider integrating the following practices into your evening routine:

1. **Breathwork**: Practice deep breathing exercises, such as diaphragmatic breathing or alternate nostril breathing, to calm the nervous system, reduce stress, and promote relaxation.
2. **Yoga**: Engage in gentle yoga postures, such as forward bends, gentle twists, and restorative poses, to release tension from the body, soothe the mind, and promote a sense of ease and well-being.
3. **Meditation**: Dedicate a few minutes to meditation or mindfulness practice to quiet the chatter of the mind, cultivate inner peace, and deepen your connection with the present moment.
4. **Herbal Tea**: Enjoy a cup of herbal tea, such as chamomile, lavender, or valerian root, to relax the body and mind, promote restful sleep, and prepare for bedtime.
5. **Warm Bath**: Take a warm bath infused with calming essential oils like lavender or sandalwood to soothe tired muscles, calm the nervous system, and induce a state of relaxation.
6. **Journaling**: Spend a few minutes journaling or reflecting on your day, expressing gratitude, and releasing any thoughts or worries that may be weighing on your mind.
7. **Digital Detox**: Power down electronic devices, such as phones, tablets, and computers, at least an hour before bedtime to minimize exposure to blue light and promote melatonin production for better sleep.

Creating an Evening Routine

Designing a personalized evening routine that incorporates calming practices before bed can help establish a sense of rhythm and ritual that signals to the body and mind that it is time to wind down and prepare for sleep. Experiment with different practices and find what works best for you, creating a nourishing and nurturing bedtime ritual that supports deep rest and rejuvenation.

As we embrace calming practices before bed and cultivate evening routines for rest, we honor the sacred transition from day to night and create space for deep relaxation, rejuvenation, and renewal. By prioritizing self-care and incorporating practices that promote relaxation and tranquility, we can create a sanctuary of peace and well-being that supports restful sleep and vibrant living. Through the transformative power of evening routines, we invite harmony and balance into our lives, nourishing body, mind, and spirit with the healing gifts of rest and renewal.

Ayurvedic Dinners: Nourishing Body and Soul

As the day draws to a close and the evening settles in, dinner takes center stage—a time to nourish the body, replenish energy stores, and promote balance and well-being. In Ayurveda, dinner holds a special significance as the final meal of the day, providing an opportunity to harmonize with the natural rhythms of the body and support optimal digestion and assimilation. In this chapter, we explore the principles of Ayurvedic dinners and how they can foster health, vitality, and harmony in our daily lives.

The Role of Dinner in Ayurveda

In Ayurveda, dinner is regarded as a pivotal meal that not only nourishes the body but also supports the process of rejuvenation and repair during sleep. As the digestive fire (Agni) naturally wanes in the evening, dinner should be lighter and easier to digest compared to the midday meal, allowing the body to focus on rest and restoration during the nighttime hours.

Principles of Ayurvedic Dinners

When planning an Ayurvedic dinner, consider the following principles to support optimal digestion, dosha balance, and overall well-being:

1. **Light and Nourishing**: Choose lighter, easily digestible foods for dinner, such as soups, steamed vegetables, grains, and legumes, to avoid burdening the digestive system and promote restful sleep.
2. **Early and Regular**: Aim to have dinner at least two to three hours before bedtime to allow ample time for digestion before sleep. Eating dinner earlier in the evening also aligns with the natural rhythms of the body and supports better sleep quality.

3. **Balanced Flavors**: Embrace a balance of flavors in your dinner, incorporating all six tastes—sweet, sour, salty, bitter, pungent, and astringent—to satisfy the palate and ensure nutritional completeness.
4. **Seasonal and Fresh**: Choose seasonal, locally sourced ingredients for your dinner to align with the rhythms of nature and maximize nutrient content and vitality. Fresh, whole foods are preferred over processed or packaged options.
5. **Mindful Eating**: Practice mindful eating during dinner, savoring each bite, chewing your food thoroughly, and eating in a calm and relaxed environment to enhance digestion and promote satisfaction.

Sample Ayurvedic Dinner Ideas

Here are a few examples of Ayurvedic dinners that you can incorporate into your meal planning:

- **Vegetable Dal with Brown Rice**: A nourishing and balanced meal featuring lentil dal cooked with seasonal vegetables and aromatic spices, served with whole grain brown rice for sustained energy and vitality.
- **Quinoa Salad with Roasted Vegetables**: A light and refreshing dinner option featuring quinoa salad with a variety of colorful vegetables, dressed with lemon-tahini dressing and garnished with fresh herbs for added flavor and nutrition.
- **Coconut Curry with Tofu and Greens**: A comforting and warming dinner choice featuring coconut curry made with tofu, mixed greens, and root vegetables, seasoned with Ayurvedic spices like turmeric, ginger, and cumin for digestive support and flavor.

Cultivating Dinner Rituals

In addition to selecting nourishing foods for dinner, consider incorporating rituals and practices that enhance the dining experience and promote connection, gratitude, and mindfulness. Lighting candles, saying a blessing or prayer, and sharing a meal with loved ones are all simple yet meaningful ways to infuse dinner time with intention and presence.

As we embrace the principles of Ayurvedic dinners and cultivate rituals that honor the sacredness of mealtime, we nourish not only our bodies but also our souls, fostering health, vitality, and harmony in every aspect of our being. By prioritizing mindful eating, seasonal ingredients, and balance in our dinner choices, we align with the wisdom of Ayurveda and create a foundation for vibrant living and holistic well-being. Through the transformative power of Ayurvedic dinners, we embark on a journey of nourishment, connection, and radiant living, guided by the ancient wisdom of Ayurveda.

Sleep Hygiene:

Cultivating Restful Nights for Vibrant Days

Sleep is a cornerstone of health and well-being—a time for the body and mind to rest, repair, and rejuvenate in preparation for the day ahead. In Ayurveda, sleep is revered as one of the three pillars of health, alongside diet and lifestyle, and is considered essential for maintaining balance and vitality. In this chapter, we explore the principles of sleep hygiene and how to cultivate restful nights for vibrant days through Ayurvedic wisdom.

Understanding Sleep in Ayurveda

In Ayurveda, sleep is viewed as a vital component of overall health and well-being, influencing physical, mental, and emotional functioning. According to Ayurvedic principles, the quality and quantity of sleep are determined by the balance of the doshas, the state of Agni (digestive fire), and the overall harmony of body and mind.

The Importance of Sleep Hygiene

Sleep hygiene refers to the habits and practices that promote restful and rejuvenating sleep, ensuring that the body and mind receive the nourishment and restoration they need to function optimally. By incorporating Ayurvedic principles into our sleep hygiene routine, we can create an environment and lifestyle that support deep, restorative sleep and enhance overall well-being.

Ayurvedic Tips for Better Sleep Hygiene

1. **Establish a Consistent Sleep Schedule**: Aim to go to bed and wake up at the same time each day, even on weekends, to regulate your body's internal clock and promote a healthy sleep-wake cycle.
2. **Create a Relaxing Bedtime Routine**: Wind down before bed with calming activities such as reading, gentle stretching, or meditation to signal to your body that it is time to relax and prepare for sleep.
3. **Create a Comfortable Sleep Environment**: Make your bedroom a sanctuary for sleep by keeping it cool, dark, and quiet. Invest in a comfortable mattress and pillows, and consider using

blackout curtains or white noise machines to block out any disturbances.
4. **Limit Screen Time Before Bed**: Minimize exposure to screens, such as phones, tablets, and computers, at least an hour before bedtime to reduce exposure to blue light, which can disrupt the production of melatonin and interfere with sleep.
5. **Avoid Heavy Meals and Stimulants Before Bed**: Refrain from consuming heavy or spicy meals, caffeine, and alcohol close to bedtime, as these can disrupt digestion and interfere with sleep quality.
6. **Practice Abhyanga (Self-Massage)**: Incorporate a nightly self-massage with warm sesame or coconut oil to relax the muscles, calm the nervous system, and promote deep relaxation before sleep.
7. **Use Herbal Remedies for Sleep Support**: Explore Ayurvedic herbs and remedies, such as ashwagandha, brahmi, and jatamansi, to support relaxation, reduce stress, and promote restful sleep.
8. **Cultivate a Mindful Sleep Mindset**: Cultivate a mindset of gratitude and relaxation as you prepare for sleep, releasing any worries or stressors from the day and inviting a sense of peace and tranquility into your mind and body.

By embracing the principles of sleep hygiene and incorporating Ayurvedic wisdom into our nightly routines, we can cultivate restful nights and vibrant days filled with energy, vitality, and well-being. Through simple yet powerful practices that honor the body's natural rhythms and support deep relaxation and rejuvenation, we tap into the transformative power of sleep and unlock the full potential of our body, mind, and spirit. As we prioritize sleep as an essential component of our daily self-care routine, we honor the sacredness of rest and embrace a life filled with health, happiness, and radiant living.

Part 3: Mind, Body, and Spirit

1. Mindful Movement:

Yoga for Your Dosha

In the timeless tradition of Ayurveda, the mind, body, and spirit are intricately connected, each influencing the other in profound ways. Mindful movement, such as yoga, serves as a powerful tool for harmonizing these aspects of our being, promoting balance, flexibility, and inner peace. In this chapter, we explore the practice of yoga through the lens of Ayurveda, offering insights into how different yoga practices can support each dosha and cultivate holistic well-being.

The Union of Yoga and Ayurveda

Yoga and Ayurveda are sister sciences, both originating from the ancient wisdom of the Vedas and sharing a common goal of promoting health, vitality, and spiritual growth. While Ayurveda focuses on the holistic healing of the body and mind through lifestyle practices, herbs, and dietary recommendations, yoga offers a path to self-awareness and self-realization through the practice of physical postures (asanas), breathwork (pranayama), and meditation (dhyana).

Understanding Your Dosha

Before diving into yoga practices tailored to each dosha, it's essential to understand the characteristics and tendencies of Vata, Pitta, and Kapha doshas:

- **Vata**: Governed by the elements of air and ether, Vata is characterized by qualities of dryness, coldness, and mobility. Vata types tend to be creative, enthusiastic, and adaptable when balanced but may experience anxiety, restlessness, and irregularity when imbalanced.
- **Pitta**: Governed by the elements of fire and water, Pitta is characterized by qualities of heat, intensity, and transformation. Pitta types tend to be ambitious, focused, and decisive when balanced but may experience anger, irritability, and inflammation when imbalanced.

- **Kapha**: Governed by the elements of earth and water, Kapha is characterized by qualities of heaviness, stability, and moisture. Kapha types tend to be compassionate, grounded, and nurturing when balanced but may experience lethargy, attachment, and congestion when imbalanced.

Yoga for Your Dosha

Tailoring your yoga practice to your dosha can help promote balance, harmony, and well-being in both body and mind. Consider the following yoga practices for each dosha:

- **Vata-Pacifying Yoga**: Vata types benefit from grounding, stabilizing yoga practices that emphasize slow, gentle movements and deep, grounding postures. Focus on hatha yoga, restorative yoga, and yin yoga to calm the nervous system, improve flexibility, and promote relaxation.
- **Pitta-Pacifying Yoga**: Pitta types benefit from cooling, calming yoga practices that help release excess heat and intensity from the body and mind. Embrace gentle, cooling practices like yin yoga, gentle flow yoga, and moon salutations to soothe the nervous system, balance emotions, and cultivate inner peace.
- **Kapha-Pacifying Yoga**: Kapha types benefit from invigorating, energizing yoga practices that stimulate circulation, promote detoxification, and awaken the body and mind. Incorporate dynamic, heating practices like vinyasa flow yoga, power yoga, and sun salutations to build heat, increase energy, and uplift the spirit.

Balancing Your Practice

Regardless of your dosha, it's essential to balance your yoga practice with elements that support overall well-being and dosha balance. Incorporate a variety of yoga styles, postures, and breathing techniques into your practice, and listen to your body's needs and limitations.

Cultivating Awareness and Intention

As you engage in mindful movement through yoga, cultivate awareness and intention in each posture and breath, connecting deeply with the present moment and the wisdom of your body. Allow your yoga practice to be a sacred journey of self-discovery and self-care, nurturing mind, body, and spirit with each mindful movement and breath.

Mindful movement through yoga offers a powerful means of harmonizing mind, body, and spirit, aligning with the ancient wisdom of Ayurveda to promote balance, vitality, and inner peace. By tailoring your yoga practice to your dosha and incorporating elements that support overall well-being, you can cultivate a deeper connection with yourself and the world around you, embracing the transformative power of yoga as a path to holistic wellness and radiant living. Through the union of yoga and Ayurveda, you embark on a journey of self-exploration and self-realization, guided by the wisdom of the ages and the innate intelligence of your body and soul.

Pranayama (Breathing Exercises)

In the intricate tapestry of yoga, the breath is revered as a bridge between the mind, body, and spirit—a sacred pathway to inner peace, vitality, and self-awareness. Pranayama, the practice of conscious breathing, offers a powerful means of cultivating mindfulness, enhancing vitality, and harmonizing the subtle energies of the body. In this chapter, we explore the transformative practice of pranayama and its profound implications for holistic well-being.

The Essence of Pranayama

Pranayama, derived from the Sanskrit words "prana" (life force) and "ayama" (extension or control), is the art of regulating the breath to balance and harmonize the flow of prana within the body. By harnessing the power of the breath, pranayama enables us to cultivate awareness, regulate energy, and connect with the deeper dimensions of our being.

The Science of Breath

In the ancient tradition of yoga, the breath is considered the primary vehicle of prana—the vital life force that animates all aspects of existence. Through conscious control of the breath, we can influence the flow of prana within the subtle energy channels (nadis) and energy centers (chakras) of the body, promoting health, vitality, and spiritual growth.

Benefits of Pranayama

The practice of pranayama offers a myriad of benefits for mind, body, and spirit, including:

- **Stress Reduction**: Pranayama techniques help calm the nervous system, reduce stress, and promote relaxation, leading to greater emotional balance and mental clarity.
- **Enhanced Vitality**: By optimizing oxygenation and circulation, pranayama increases energy levels, improves stamina, and enhances overall vitality and well-being.
- **Improved Respiratory Health**: Pranayama strengthens the respiratory muscles, increases lung capacity, and promotes efficient breathing, supporting respiratory health and function.
- **Balanced Energy**: Through pranayama, we can regulate the flow of prana and balance the subtle energies of the body, fostering a sense of equilibrium and inner harmony.

Pranayama Techniques for Mindful Movement

Here are a few foundational pranayama techniques to incorporate into your mindful movement practice:

1. **Dirga Swasam (Three-Part Breath)**: Begin by inhaling deeply into the abdomen, then expanding the ribcage, and finally filling the chest with breath. Exhale slowly and fully, releasing the breath from the chest, ribcage, and abdomen in succession. Repeat for several rounds, focusing on smooth, even breaths.
2. **Nadi Shodhana (Alternate Nostril Breathing)**: Close the right nostril with the right thumb and inhale deeply through the left nostril. Close the left nostril with the right ring finger, exhale through the right nostril, then inhale through the right nostril. Close the right nostril again and exhale through the left nostril. Repeat for several rounds, alternating nostrils with each breath.
3. **Sitali Pranayama (Cooling Breath)**: Curl the sides of the tongue to form a tube-like shape. Inhale deeply through the curled tongue, allowing the breath to cool the body. Exhale slowly through the nose. Continue for several rounds, focusing on the sensation of coolness with each inhalation.

Cultivating Awareness and Presence

As you engage in pranayama practice, cultivate mindfulness and presence with each breath, anchoring your awareness in the present moment and the rhythmic flow of the breath. Notice any sensations, thoughts, or emotions that arise without judgment, allowing them to come and go like waves on the ocean of consciousness.

Integrating Pranayama into Daily Life

Beyond the confines of the yoga mat, pranayama can be integrated into daily life as a tool for cultivating mindfulness, reducing stress, and enhancing well-being. Whether you're sitting in traffic, waiting in line, or navigating a challenging situation, the breath is always available as a source of grounding and centering.

In the practice of pranayama, we tap into the transformative power of the breath—a sacred pathway to inner peace, vitality, and self-awareness. By cultivating mindfulness and presence with each inhalation and exhalation, we awaken to the fullness of life and the infinite potential within ourselves. Through the practice of pranayama, we embark on a journey of self-discovery and self-realization, guided by the wisdom of the breath and the boundless expanse of our own inner landscape.

Meditation Techniques:

Cultivating Stillness in the Midst of Movement

In the fast-paced modern world, where distractions abound and demands constantly vie for our attention, meditation serves as a sanctuary of stillness—a refuge where we can anchor ourselves in the present moment and reconnect with the essence of our being. In this chapter, we explore a variety of meditation techniques drawn from the ancient wisdom of Ayurveda and other contemplative traditions, offering practical guidance for cultivating inner peace, clarity, and presence in our daily lives.

The Essence of Meditation

Meditation is a practice of mindfulness and self-awareness—a journey inward to explore the depths of our consciousness and awaken to the innate wisdom and tranquility that reside within us. Rooted in the timeless wisdom of ancient traditions such as Ayurveda, yoga, Buddhism, and

Taoism, meditation offers a pathway to inner peace, insight, and spiritual growth.

Types of Meditation Techniques

There are countless meditation techniques, each offering a unique approach to cultivating mindfulness, concentration, and inner peace. Here are a few widely practiced techniques to explore:

1. **Mindfulness Meditation**: In mindfulness meditation, we cultivate present-moment awareness by observing the breath, bodily sensations, thoughts, and emotions with non-judgmental awareness. By anchoring our attention in the present moment, we develop clarity, acceptance, and equanimity.
2. **Mantra Meditation**: Mantra meditation involves repeating a sacred word, phrase, or sound (mantra) silently or aloud to focus the mind and transcend ordinary consciousness. Mantras can be traditional Sanskrit chants, affirmations, or personal intentions that resonate with the practitioner's heart.
3. **Loving-Kindness Meditation (Metta)**: Loving-kindness meditation cultivates compassion, empathy, and unconditional love by directing well-wishes and blessings towards oneself, loved ones, neutral individuals, and even difficult people. This practice fosters a sense of interconnectedness and universal goodwill.
4. **Visualization (Guided Imagery)**: Visualization meditation involves mentally picturing specific images, scenes, or symbols to evoke feelings of relaxation, healing, and empowerment. Guided imagery scripts may lead practitioners through peaceful landscapes, healing journeys, or encounters with inner guides.
5. **Breath Awareness (Pranayama)**: Breath awareness meditation focuses on observing the natural rhythm of the breath as it flows in and out of the body. By anchoring our attention in the breath, we cultivate presence, calmness, and inner stillness.

Cultivating a Meditation Practice

Whether you're a seasoned meditator or just beginning your journey, cultivating a regular meditation practice requires commitment, patience, and self-compassion. Here are some tips for establishing and sustaining a meditation practice:

- **Start Small**: Begin with just a few minutes of meditation each day and gradually increase the duration as you become more comfortable and confident in your practice.
- **Find a Quiet Space**: Create a dedicated meditation space in your home where you can sit comfortably and without distractions. This could be a corner of a room, a cushion on the floor, or a special chair.
- **Establish a Routine**: Incorporate meditation into your daily routine by practicing at the same time each day, whether it's upon waking, during your lunch break, or before bed.
- **Experiment with Different Techniques**: Explore different meditation techniques to find what resonates with you. Remember that there is no one-size-fits-all approach, and it's okay to experiment and adapt your practice over time.
- **Be Gentle with Yourself**: Approach meditation with an attitude of kindness, curiosity, and non-judgment. Be patient with yourself as you navigate the ups and downs of the practice, and celebrate your progress along the way.

Integrating Meditation into Daily Life

Beyond formal meditation sessions, meditation can be integrated into daily life as a way of cultivating mindfulness and presence in every moment. Whether you're walking, eating, or engaging in daily activities, you can bring a spirit of awareness and attentiveness to your experience, infusing even the most mundane tasks with a sense of sacredness and reverence.

In the practice of meditation, we embark on a journey of self-discovery and self-transformation—a journey that leads us inward to the depths of our own being. Through the cultivation of mindfulness, concentration, and inner stillness, we awaken to the timeless wisdom that resides within us, unlocking the door to peace, clarity, and fulfillment. As we embrace meditation as a daily practice, we open ourselves to the infinite possibilities of the present moment, tapping into the boundless reservoir of peace and joy that lies at the heart of our true nature.

2. Ayurvedic Self-Care:

Skin and Hair Care Routines

In the ancient tradition of Ayurveda, self-care is regarded as an essential practice for promoting health, vitality, and well-being on all levels—physical, mental, and spiritual. By cultivating self-awareness, self-compassion, and self-love, we honor the sacred vessel of our body and soul, nurturing radiance from within. In this chapter, we explore Ayurvedic self-care rituals for skin and hair, offering time-honored practices to support beauty, vitality, and holistic wellness.

The Art of Ayurvedic Self-Care

Ayurvedic self-care is rooted in the principle of holistic wellness—a philosophy that recognizes the interconnectedness of mind, body, and spirit. By integrating self-care practices into our daily routines, we honor the unique needs of our body and soul, fostering harmony, balance, and vitality in every aspect of our being.

Skin Care Rituals

The skin is the body's largest organ, serving as a protective barrier between the internal and external environments. Ayurveda views the skin as a reflection of our inner health and vitality, emphasizing the importance of nurturing and nourishing the skin to maintain its natural beauty and radiance. Here are some Ayurvedic skin care rituals to incorporate into your daily routine:

1. **Abhyanga (Self-Massage)**: Begin your day with a nourishing self-massage using warm sesame, coconut, or almond oil. Massage the entire body in gentle, circular motions, paying special attention to areas of tension or dryness. Abhyanga not only hydrates the skin but also promotes relaxation, circulation, and detoxification.
2. **Herbal Cleansing**: Cleanse the skin with gentle, natural ingredients such as chickpea flour (besan), rose water, or herbal powders like neem or turmeric. These traditional Ayurvedic

cleansers help remove impurities, balance oil production, and promote a clear, radiant complexion.
3. **Hydration**: Hydrate the skin from within by drinking plenty of water throughout the day to maintain moisture balance and support detoxification. Additionally, apply a hydrating moisturizer or herbal oil to the skin after bathing to lock in moisture and protect against environmental stressors.
4. **Facial Steaming**: Incorporate facial steaming into your weekly routine to cleanse pores, remove impurities, and promote circulation. Add Ayurvedic herbs such as lavender, rose petals, or chamomile to the steaming water for added benefits.
5. **Sun Protection**: Protect the skin from harmful UV rays by wearing sunscreen or natural sun protection products containing ingredients like zinc oxide or titanium dioxide. Additionally, seek shade during peak sun hours and wear protective clothing when outdoors.

Hair Care Rituals

In Ayurveda, the hair is considered a reflection of overall health and vitality, requiring nourishment and care to maintain strength, luster, and vitality. Ayurvedic hair care rituals focus on promoting healthy hair growth, soothing the scalp, and maintaining balance in the hair and scalp ecosystem. Here are some Ayurvedic hair care practices to incorporate into your routine:

1. **Scalp Massage**: Massage the scalp regularly with warm oil, such as coconut, almond, or Brahmi oil, to nourish the hair follicles, improve circulation, and soothe the scalp. Use gentle, circular motions to distribute the oil evenly and leave it on for at least 30 minutes before shampooing.
2. **Herbal Hair Wash**: Wash your hair with gentle, natural cleansers such as shikakai, reetha (soapnut), or amla (Indian gooseberry) to cleanse the scalp and hair without stripping away natural oils. These Ayurvedic herbs help maintain pH balance, reduce dandruff, and promote healthy hair growth.
3. **Nutritive Hair Masks**: Treat your hair to nourishing hair masks made from Ayurvedic ingredients such as yogurt, aloe vera, fenugreek, or hibiscus. These natural ingredients help condition the hair, strengthen the roots, and add shine and vitality to your locks.

4. **Scalp Exfoliation**: Exfoliate the scalp regularly to remove dead skin cells, excess oil, and product buildup, which can clog pores and inhibit healthy hair growth. Use a gentle scalp scrub made from ingredients like sea salt, brown sugar, or finely ground oats to promote a clean, healthy scalp.
5. **Healthy Lifestyle Habits**: Support healthy hair from the inside out by maintaining a balanced diet, staying hydrated, managing stress, and getting regular exercise. A holistic approach to wellness promotes overall vitality, which is reflected in the health and beauty of your hair.

Ayurvedic self-care rituals for skin and hair offer a holistic approach to beauty and wellness, honoring the interconnectedness of mind, body, and spirit. By incorporating these time-honored practices into your daily routine, you can nurture radiance from within, promoting health, vitality, and holistic well-being on all levels. As you embark on your journey of self-care, remember to cultivate self-awareness, self-compassion, and self-love, embracing the sacredness of your body and soul with every nourishing ritual and loving gesture.

Ayurvedic Beauty Secrets:

Radiant Glow from Within

In the timeless tradition of Ayurveda, beauty is regarded as an expression of inner health, vitality, and balance—a reflection of the harmonious interplay of mind, body, and spirit. Ayurvedic beauty secrets offer a holistic approach to skincare, embracing natural ingredients, mindful practices, and self-care rituals to promote a radiant glow from within. In this chapter, we delve into the ancient wisdom of Ayurveda to uncover the secrets to lasting beauty and timeless elegance.

The Essence of Ayurvedic Beauty

Ayurvedic beauty is rooted in the principle of holistic wellness—a philosophy that recognizes the interconnectedness of physical, mental, and spiritual aspects of being. According to Ayurveda, true beauty emanates from inner harmony, balance, and vitality, manifesting as a radiant glow that transcends external appearances.

Ayurvedic Principles for Beautiful Skin

In Ayurveda, beautiful skin is seen as a reflection of overall health and well-being, requiring nourishment, hydration, and balance from within. By embracing Ayurvedic principles for skincare, we can support the natural beauty and radiance of our skin. Here are some Ayurvedic beauty secrets for healthy, glowing skin:

1. **Balancing Doshas**: According to Ayurveda, imbalances in the doshas (Vata, Pitta, and Kapha) can manifest as skin issues such as dryness, inflammation, or congestion. Tailor your skincare routine to your dominant dosha to restore balance and harmony to the skin.
2. **Nourishing Oils**: Ayurvedic oils such as sesame, coconut, and almond are revered for their hydrating, nourishing properties. Incorporate daily self-massage (Abhyanga) with warm oil to moisturize the skin, improve circulation, and promote a healthy glow.
3. **Herbal Cleansing**: Cleanse the skin with gentle, natural ingredients such as chickpea flour (besan), rose water, or herbal powders like neem or turmeric. These traditional Ayurvedic cleansers help remove impurities, balance oil production, and promote a clear, radiant complexion.
4. **Hydration**: Hydrate the skin from within by drinking plenty of water throughout the day to maintain moisture balance and support detoxification. Additionally, apply a hydrating moisturizer or herbal oil to the skin after bathing to lock in moisture and protect against environmental stressors.
5. **Nutrient-Rich Diet**: Support skin health by eating a balanced diet rich in nutrients, antioxidants, and essential fatty acids. Incorporate foods such as fresh fruits and vegetables, whole grains, nuts, seeds, and healthy fats to nourish the skin from the inside out.

Ayurvedic Secrets for Lustrous Hair

In Ayurveda, hair is seen as a symbol of vitality and vitality, requiring nourishment, care, and attention to maintain strength, luster, and shine. Here are some Ayurvedic beauty secrets for healthy, lustrous hair:

1. **Scalp Massage**: Massage the scalp regularly with warm oil, such as coconut, almond, or Brahmi oil, to nourish the hair follicles, improve circulation, and soothe the scalp. Use gentle, circular motions to distribute the oil evenly and leave it on for at least 30 minutes before shampooing.
2. **Herbal Hair Wash**: Wash your hair with gentle, natural cleansers such as shikakai, reetha (soapnut), or amla (Indian gooseberry) to cleanse the scalp and hair without stripping away natural oils. These Ayurvedic herbs help maintain pH balance, reduce dandruff, and promote healthy hair growth.
3. **Nutritive Hair Masks**: Treat your hair to nourishing hair masks made from Ayurvedic ingredients such as yogurt, aloe vera, fenugreek, or hibiscus. These natural ingredients help condition the hair, strengthen the roots, and add shine and vitality to your locks.
4. **Scalp Exfoliation**: Exfoliate the scalp regularly to remove dead skin cells, excess oil, and product buildup, which can clog pores and inhibit healthy hair growth. Use a gentle scalp scrub made from ingredients like sea salt, brown sugar, or finely ground oats to promote a clean, healthy scalp.
5. **Healthy Lifestyle Habits**: Support healthy hair from the inside out by maintaining a balanced diet, staying hydrated, managing stress, and getting regular exercise. A holistic approach to wellness promotes overall vitality, which is reflected in the health and beauty of your hair.

Cultivating Inner Radiance

Beyond external beauty, Ayurvedic self-care invites us to cultivate inner radiance—a deep sense of self-love, acceptance, and appreciation for the beauty that resides within us. By embracing Ayurvedic beauty secrets and nurturing our body, mind, and spirit with love and care, we awaken to the timeless beauty and grace that is our birthright.

Ayurvedic beauty secrets offer a holistic approach to skincare and haircare, honoring the interconnectedness of mind, body, and spirit. By incorporating these time-honored practices into your daily routine, you can nourish your skin, hair, and soul, promoting a radiant glow from within. As you embark on your journey of Ayurvedic self-care, remember to cultivate self-love, self-compassion, and self-acceptance, embracing the beauty and uniqueness of your being with every loving gesture and nurturing ritual.

Self-Massage Techniques for Nurturing Body and Soul

In the ancient tradition of Ayurveda, self-care is regarded as a sacred practice—an opportunity to honor and nurture the body, mind, and spirit with love and compassion. Self-massage, known as Abhyanga, is a cornerstone of Ayurvedic self-care, offering a powerful means of promoting relaxation, vitality, and holistic well-being. In this chapter, we explore the art of self-massage and share time-honored techniques for nurturing body and soul.

The Healing Power of Self-Massage

Self-massage, or Abhyanga, is a practice of self-care and self-love that dates back thousands of years in Ayurvedic tradition. Derived from the Sanskrit words "abhi" (towards) and "anga" (limb), Abhyanga involves massaging warm oil into the skin to nourish the tissues, calm the nervous system, and promote a sense of deep relaxation and well-being.

Benefits of Self-Massage

The practice of self-massage offers a myriad of benefits for physical, mental, and emotional health, including:

- **Nourishing the Skin**: Massage helps improve circulation, promote lymphatic drainage, and enhance the absorption of nutrients, leaving the skin soft, supple, and glowing.
- **Relieving Stress and Tension**: The rhythmic movements of massage soothe the nervous system, release muscular tension, and induce a state of deep relaxation, reducing stress and anxiety.
- **Supporting Detoxification**: Massage stimulates the lymphatic system, helping to remove toxins and waste products from the body and support overall detoxification.
- **Balancing the Doshas**: Abhyanga helps balance the doshas (Vata, Pitta, and Kapha) by calming Vata, cooling Pitta, and

invigorating Kapha, promoting harmony and balance in body and mind.

Self-Massage Techniques

To perform self-massage, follow these simple steps:

1. **Choose Your Oil**: Select a high-quality oil that is appropriate for your dosha or the season. Popular choices include sesame oil for Vata, coconut oil for Pitta, and mustard oil for Kapha.
2. **Warm the Oil**: Place the oil in a container and warm it gently by placing the container in a bowl of warm water. Alternatively, you can warm the oil by rubbing it between your palms.
3. **Prepare Your Space**: Find a quiet, comfortable space where you can perform your self-massage undisturbed. Lay down a towel or old sheet to protect your clothing and surroundings.
4. **Begin at the Feet**: Start by massaging your feet with long, sweeping strokes, working from the toes towards the ankles. Use circular motions to massage the soles of the feet, paying special attention to any areas of tension or discomfort.
5. **Move Upwards**: Gradually work your way up the body, massaging each limb with long, rhythmic strokes. Use circular motions to massage the joints (knees, elbows, shoulders) and smaller circular motions to massage the abdomen and chest.
6. **Focus on the Head and Scalp**: Finish your self-massage by massaging your head and scalp with gentle, circular motions. Pay special attention to the temples, forehead, and the base of the skull, where tension often accumulates.
7. **Rest and Rejuvenate**: After completing your self-massage, take a few moments to rest and allow the oil to penetrate the skin. You can wrap yourself in a warm towel or relax in a warm bath to enhance the effects of the massage.

Cultivating Self-Love and Compassion

As you engage in the practice of self-massage, cultivate a spirit of self-love, self-compassion, and self-acceptance. Approach your body with kindness and gratitude, honoring its wisdom and resilience. Allow the healing power of touch to nourish and rejuvenate your body, mind, and spirit, fostering a deep sense of connection and wholeness.

Self-massage is a sacred practice of self-care and self-love—a time-honored tradition that nourishes body and soul with love and compassion. By incorporating self-massage into your daily routine, you can promote relaxation, vitality, and holistic well-being on all levels. As you embrace the healing power of touch, remember to cultivate a spirit of self-love, self-compassion, and self-acceptance, honoring the sacred vessel of your body with every nurturing gesture and loving touch.

3. Ayurvedic Healing

Common Ayurvedic Remedies

In the realm of Ayurveda, healing is a holistic journey that encompasses the body, mind, and spirit. Rooted in ancient wisdom, Ayurvedic remedies offer a treasure trove of natural solutions to address various ailments and imbalances. From herbs and spices to lifestyle practices and dietary adjustments, Ayurveda provides a comprehensive approach to promoting health and well-being. In this chapter, we delve into some of the most common Ayurvedic remedies that have stood the test of time, offering insights into their therapeutic properties and applications.

1. Triphala: Known as the "nectar of life," Triphala is a powerful herbal concoction comprised of three fruits: Amalaki (Emblica officinalis), Bibhitaki (Terminalia bellirica), and Haritaki (Terminalia chebula). This tridoshic formula serves as a gentle yet effective cleanser for the digestive system, promoting regularity, detoxification, and rejuvenation. Triphala also supports healthy digestion, absorption, and assimilation of nutrients, making it a cornerstone remedy in Ayurvedic practice.

2. Ashwagandha: Revered as the "Indian ginseng," Ashwagandha is an adaptogenic herb renowned for its ability to combat stress and promote vitality. Withania somnifera, the botanical name for Ashwagandha, helps the body adapt to physical, mental, and emotional stressors, thereby enhancing resilience and overall well-being. This rejuvenating herb also supports healthy adrenal function, boosts immunity, and fosters a sense of calm and balance in the mind.

3. Turmeric: A golden-hued spice prized for its medicinal properties, turmeric (Curcuma longa) has been a cornerstone of Ayurvedic healing for millennia. Curcumin, the active compound in turmeric, exhibits potent anti-inflammatory, antioxidant, and antimicrobial effects, making it a versatile remedy for a myriad of health concerns. From alleviating joint pain and supporting digestive health to enhancing cognitive function and promoting radiant skin, turmeric is a true powerhouse in Ayurvedic medicine.

4. Tulsi (Holy Basil): Revered as the "Queen of Herbs" in Ayurveda, Tulsi (Ocimum sanctum) holds a sacred place in Indian culture and traditional medicine. This aromatic herb boasts a wide array of therapeutic properties, including adaptogenic, immune-enhancing, and stress-relieving effects. Tulsi is renowned for its ability to purify the mind, body, and spirit, promoting clarity, vitality, and inner harmony. Whether consumed as a tea, tincture, or fresh leaves, Tulsi serves as a potent ally for holistic health and well-being.

5. Ghee: In Ayurveda, ghee (clarified butter) is revered as a potent elixir with rejuvenating properties. Rich in essential fatty acids, vitamins, and antioxidants, ghee nourishes the body at a cellular level, promoting strength, vitality, and longevity. This golden substance is also prized for its ability to pacify Vata and Pitta doshas, making it a valuable therapeutic remedy for individuals seeking balance and stability. Whether used internally or externally, ghee serves as a cornerstone of Ayurvedic healing, fostering health and vitality from within.

6. Trikatu: Translating to "three pungents," Trikatu is a potent herbal formula comprised of equal parts ginger (Zingiber officinale), black pepper (Piper nigrum), and long pepper (Piper longum). This fiery blend ignites the digestive fire (agni), promoting healthy metabolism, assimilation, and elimination. Trikatu is particularly beneficial for individuals with sluggish digestion, poor appetite, or respiratory congestion, offering warmth, stimulation, and clarity to the body and mind.

7. Neem: Dubbed the "village pharmacy" in India, neem (Azadirachta indica) is a versatile botanical renowned for its potent antibacterial, antifungal, and antiviral properties. Neem is traditionally used to purify the blood, support immune function, and promote skin health, making it a valuable remedy for a variety of ailments. Whether applied topically or taken internally, neem serves as a potent ally for detoxification, protection, and rejuvenation, embodying the essence of Ayurvedic healing.

Ayurvedic remedies offer a holistic approach to health and well-being, addressing the root causes of imbalance while nurturing the body's innate capacity for healing. From herbs and spices to dietary principles and lifestyle practices, Ayurveda provides a comprehensive toolkit for promoting vitality, longevity, and radiant health. By integrating these ancient wisdom traditions into our modern lives, we can cultivate greater harmony, resilience, and vitality in body, mind, and spirit.

Detoxification and Panchakarma

In the journey toward optimal health and well-being, detoxification plays a pivotal role in Ayurvedic healing. Rooted in the ancient wisdom of India, Ayurveda recognizes the importance of periodically cleansing the body and mind to remove accumulated toxins, rejuvenate the tissues, and restore balance to the doshas. At the heart of Ayurvedic detoxification lies Panchakarma, a comprehensive cleansing and rejuvenation protocol designed to purify the body on a deep level. In this chapter, we explore the principles of Ayurvedic detoxification and the transformative power of Panchakarma.

Ayurvedic Healing Through Detoxification:

Ayurveda views health as a state of dynamic equilibrium between the doshas (Vata, Pitta, and Kapha), agni (digestive fire), and the dhatus (tissues) of the body. When the natural balance is disturbed due to poor dietary habits, environmental toxins, stress, or other factors, toxins known as ama accumulate in the body, disrupting cellular function and leading to disease.

Detoxification in Ayurveda aims to eliminate ama and restore balance to the doshas, allowing the body to function optimally. This process involves a combination of dietary modifications, herbal therapies, lifestyle practices, and cleansing techniques tailored to individual constitution and imbalances.

Key Principles of Ayurvedic Detoxification:

1. **Agni Kindling**: Central to Ayurvedic detoxification is the cultivation of strong agni, or digestive fire. Ama arises from poorly digested food due to weak agni, so enhancing digestive function is essential for effective detoxification. This can be achieved through the consumption of warming spices, such as ginger, cumin, and black pepper, which stimulate agni and facilitate the digestion and elimination of toxins.
2. **Purification Therapies**: Ayurveda offers a variety of purification therapies, or shodhana, to cleanse the body of accumulated toxins. These may include fasting, herbal teas, oil massage (abhyanga), herbal enemas (basti), nasal cleansing (nasya), and tongue scraping. These practices help to eliminate impurities from the digestive tract, lymphatic system, and other bodily tissues, promoting detoxification and rejuvenation.
3. **Dietary Cleansing**: Dietary modifications are an integral part of Ayurvedic detoxification. During a cleanse, emphasis is placed on consuming light, easily digestible foods such as whole grains, steamed vegetables, soups, and herbal teas. Avoidance of processed foods, refined sugars, caffeine, alcohol, and heavy meats is recommended to support the body's natural detoxification processes.
4. **Mind-Body Practices**: Detoxification in Ayurveda is not limited to the physical body but also encompasses the mind and emotions. Practices such as meditation, pranayama (breathwork), yoga, and mindfulness help to calm the mind, reduce stress, and promote mental clarity, facilitating the release of emotional toxins and promoting overall well-being.

Panchakarma: The Ayurvedic Detoxification Protocol:

Panchakarma is the crown jewel of Ayurvedic detoxification, offering a comprehensive and systematic approach to cleansing and rejuvenation. Translating to "five actions" in Sanskrit, Panchakarma consists of five main therapeutic modalities designed to purify the body on a deep level:

1. **Vamana (Therapeutic Emesis)**: Vamana involves the administration of emetic substances to induce controlled vomiting, expelling excess Kapha dosha and toxins from the upper respiratory tract and stomach.

2. **Virechana (Therapeutic Purgation)**: Virechana entails the use of purgative herbs to stimulate bowel movements and eliminate excess Pitta dosha and toxins from the intestines and liver.
3. **Basti (Therapeutic Enema)**: Basti involves the administration of medicated enemas to cleanse the colon and balance Vata dosha. Basti nourishes and lubricates the tissues while removing accumulated toxins and ama.
4. **Nasya (Nasal Administration)**: Nasya involves the application of medicated oils or herbal preparations to the nasal passages to cleanse and purify the sinuses, respiratory tract, and brain.
5. **Rakta Mokshana (Bloodletting Therapy)**: Rakta Mokshana is a specialized technique used to purify the blood and remove excess Pitta dosha and toxins from the body.

Panchakarma is typically conducted under the guidance of a trained Ayurvedic practitioner and customized to individual needs and imbalances. The process begins with a preparatory phase to prepare the body for cleansing, followed by the main detoxification therapies, and concludes with a rejuvenation phase to nourish and rebuild the tissues.

Ayurvedic detoxification is a time-honored practice that offers profound healing and rejuvenation for body, mind, and spirit. By incorporating principles of purification into our daily lives and undergoing periodic Panchakarma treatments, we can support the body's innate ability to detoxify and restore balance, fostering optimal health and vitality in the modern world.

Managing Stress and Anxiety

In the fast-paced world of modern living, stress and anxiety have become ubiquitous companions for many. Fortunately, Ayurveda offers a wealth of wisdom and practices to help manage and alleviate these common afflictions. Rooted in ancient teachings, Ayurvedic healing approaches stress and anxiety from a holistic perspective, addressing imbalances in body, mind, and spirit. In this chapter, we explore the principles and practices of Ayurveda for managing stress and anxiety, offering actionable insights for cultivating greater peace, resilience, and well-being in daily life.

Understanding Stress and Anxiety in Ayurveda:

According to Ayurveda, stress and anxiety arise from imbalances in the doshas (Vata, Pitta, and Kapha), as well as disturbances in the mind (manas) and emotions (manasika). When the doshas are out of harmony or when the mind is agitated, individuals may experience symptoms such as restlessness, worry, insomnia, irritability, and fatigue.

Ayurveda recognizes that stress and anxiety are multifaceted conditions that require a comprehensive approach to healing. Rather than simply masking symptoms, Ayurvedic healing seeks to address the underlying imbalances and restore equilibrium to the body and mind.

Key Principles of Ayurvedic Healing for Stress and Anxiety:

1. **Balancing the Doshas**: Central to Ayurvedic healing for stress and anxiety is the restoration of balance to the doshas. Depending on individual constitution and imbalances, different strategies may be employed to pacify aggravated doshas and promote harmony. For example, individuals with excess Vata may benefit from grounding practices and nourishing foods, while those with excess Pitta may benefit from cooling and calming therapies.
2. **Nurturing Ojas**: In Ayurveda, ojas is the subtle essence of vitality, immunity, and resilience. Chronic stress and anxiety deplete ojas, leaving individuals feeling depleted and susceptible to illness. Ayurvedic practices that nourish ojas include consuming wholesome foods, engaging in self-care rituals, and cultivating positive emotions such as love, compassion, and gratitude.

3. **Strengthening Agni**: Ayurveda teaches that strong agni, or digestive fire, is essential for optimal health and vitality. When agni is weak, undigested food (ama) accumulates in the body, leading to physical and mental imbalances. Strengthening agni through dietary adjustments, herbal remedies, and lifestyle practices helps to promote efficient digestion and metabolism, supporting overall well-being.
4. **Practicing Mindfulness**: Mindfulness is a cornerstone of Ayurvedic healing for stress and anxiety. By cultivating present-moment awareness and non-judgmental observation of thoughts and sensations, individuals can reduce stress reactivity and cultivate inner peace. Mindfulness practices such as meditation, breathwork (pranayama), and yoga help to calm the mind, balance the nervous system, and promote relaxation.
5. **Herbal Therapies**: Ayurveda offers a rich pharmacopoeia of herbs and botanicals renowned for their calming and adaptogenic properties. Adaptogens such as ashwagandha, brahmi (gotu kola), and shatavari help the body adapt to stress and promote resilience, while nervine herbs such as chamomile, lavender, and passionflower soothe the nervous system and support emotional balance.

Practical Tips for Managing Stress and Anxiety:

- Establish a daily routine (dinacharya) that includes regular sleep, meals, exercise, and relaxation.
- Prioritize self-care activities such as massage, aromatherapy, and spending time in nature.
- Cultivate supportive relationships and seek guidance from trusted mentors or practitioners.
- Limit exposure to stressors such as excessive screen time, caffeine, and stimulating media.
- Practice gratitude, compassion, and forgiveness to foster a positive outlook and emotional resilience.

Ayurveda offers a holistic approach to managing stress and anxiety, addressing imbalances in body, mind, and spirit. By incorporating Ayurvedic principles and practices into daily life, individuals can cultivate greater peace, resilience, and well-being, even in the midst of life's challenges. Through nurturing the doshas, nurturing ojas, strengthening agni, practicing mindfulness, and utilizing herbal therapies, we can harness the ancient wisdom of Ayurveda to navigate the complexities of modern living with grace and equanimity.

4. Seasonal Ayurveda

Adapting Practices with the Seasons

Ayurveda, the ancient system of medicine from India, emphasizes harmony with nature and its cycles. Central to Ayurvedic philosophy is the understanding that our well-being is profoundly affected by the changing seasons. Each season brings its unique qualities, which can either support or challenge our health. By aligning our lifestyle, diet, and practices with the rhythms of nature, we can maintain balance and promote optimal health throughout the year. This chapter delves into the principles of seasonal Ayurveda, providing guidance on how to adapt our routines to the cycles of Vata, Pitta, and Kapha doshas.

Spring (Kapha Season)

Spring is a time of renewal and growth, associated with the Kapha dosha, which embodies the qualities of earth and water. The lingering cold and dampness of winter give way to a moist, heavy, and cool environment. During this period, it's common to experience Kapha imbalances such as colds, congestion, and sluggishness. To counteract these effects, Ayurveda recommends practices that are invigorating and lightening.

Dietary adjustments in spring should focus on foods that are warm, light, and dry to help balance the heavy and moist nature of Kapha. Emphasize bitter, pungent, and astringent tastes while reducing sweet, sour, and salty flavors. Incorporate more green vegetables, legumes, and spices like ginger, turmeric, and black pepper, which aid digestion and reduce congestion.

Physical activity is essential in spring to invigorate the body and mind. Engage in dynamic exercises like jogging, cycling, or dancing to stimulate circulation and dispel lethargy. Morning routines can include dry brushing and oil massage with invigorating oils such as mustard or sesame, followed by a warm shower to enhance circulation and detoxification.

Summer (Pitta Season)

Summer, governed by the Pitta dosha, is characterized by heat, intensity, and transformation. The rising temperatures and longer days can exacerbate Pitta-related issues such as overheating, inflammation, and irritability. To maintain balance during the summer, it is crucial to adopt cooling, soothing, and hydrating practices.

A Pitta-pacifying diet includes foods that are cool, sweet, and mildly astringent. Fresh fruits like melons, grapes, and berries, as well as vegetables like cucumbers, zucchini, and leafy greens, are ideal. Avoid excessively spicy, salty, and sour foods, which can increase internal heat. Incorporate herbs such as mint, coriander, and fennel, which have cooling properties.

Hydration is vital during the summer months. Drink plenty of water, herbal teas, and coconut water to stay hydrated and cool. Avoid caffeine and alcohol, which can be dehydrating and overheating.

Physical activities should be moderate and performed during the cooler parts of the day, such as early morning or late evening. Swimming, walking, and gentle yoga are excellent choices to keep the body fit without generating excess heat. Incorporate cooling practices into your daily routine, such as applying aloe vera gel or sandalwood paste to the skin and taking cool showers.

Autumn (Vata Season)

Autumn is marked by the predominance of the Vata dosha, which brings qualities of dryness, lightness, and mobility. The transition from the warmth of summer to the coolness of winter can lead to Vata imbalances, manifesting as dry skin, anxiety, and irregular digestion. To ground and nourish Vata during this season, focus on warmth, stability, and moisture.

A Vata-pacifying diet includes warm, cooked, and moist foods with sweet, sour, and salty tastes. Emphasize root vegetables, grains, and dairy products, and incorporate warming spices like cinnamon, cardamom, and cloves. Soups, stews, and casseroles are excellent choices to provide warmth and sustenance.

Routine and regularity are essential to counteract the erratic nature of Vata. Establish consistent daily routines for eating, sleeping, and working to provide stability. Warm oil massages using sesame or almond oil can help to moisturize the skin and calm the nervous system. Engage in calming exercises like yoga, tai chi, or walking to maintain physical and mental balance.

Winter (Vata-Kapha Season)

Winter is a complex season where both Vata and Kapha doshas play a role. Early winter tends to be more Vata-like, while late winter takes on Kapha characteristics. The cold, heavy, and damp environment can challenge both doshas, requiring a balanced approach to maintain harmony.

During early winter, continue with the warm, moist, and nourishing practices suitable for Vata. As the season progresses, and Kapha becomes more dominant, adjust the diet to include more light and spicy foods to prevent Kapha buildup. Ginger tea, warm soups, and hearty grains like quinoa and millet are beneficial throughout winter.

Physical activity should be regular and stimulating to counter the sluggishness of Kapha and the instability of Vata. Brisk walking, strength training, and aerobic exercises can help keep the body warm and energized. Indoor activities can be particularly beneficial when the weather is harsh.

Practicing mindfulness and staying connected with loved ones can also help counter the seasonal blues often associated with winter. Engage in hobbies and social activities that bring joy and warmth to the heart.

By understanding the interplay of doshas and seasons, Ayurveda provides a framework for living in harmony with the natural world. Adapting our diets, routines, and activities to the changing seasons helps maintain balance, prevent illness, and promote overall well-being. Embracing these practices allows us to thrive in sync with the rhythms of nature, embodying the wisdom of Ayurveda in our daily lives.

Seasonal Diet and Lifestyle Tips

Ayurveda, the ancient Indian system of holistic health, teaches us to live in harmony with the natural rhythms of the environment. One of the foundational principles of Ayurveda is aligning our diet and lifestyle with the changing seasons to maintain balance and health. Each season brings specific qualities that influence our physical and mental well-being. By understanding and adapting to these seasonal shifts, we can enhance our vitality and prevent imbalances that lead to illness.

Spring, associated with the Kapha dosha, is a season of renewal and growth. The environment becomes moist, heavy, and cool as the coldness of winter melts away. This can lead to an accumulation of Kapha in the body, causing issues like congestion, allergies, and lethargy. To counteract these effects, Ayurveda recommends a light, dry, and warming diet to balance Kapha's heavy and moist qualities. Incorporate more bitter, pungent, and astringent tastes into your meals. Fresh greens, sprouts, and a variety of spices such as turmeric, ginger, and black pepper are ideal. Avoid dairy, cold foods, and anything overly sweet or salty, as these can increase Kapha. Lifestyle practices should focus on invigorating activities. Start your day with a brisk walk or a vigorous yoga session to stimulate circulation and dispel sluggishness. Dry brushing and using light, stimulating oils like mustard or sesame for self-massage can further invigorate your system.

Summer is ruled by the Pitta dosha, characterized by heat, intensity, and brightness. The rising temperatures and longer days can aggravate Pitta, leading to issues like overheating, irritability, and inflammation. To keep Pitta in check, embrace a diet that is cool, light, and hydrating. Favor sweet, bitter, and astringent tastes, which have a cooling effect on the body. Fresh fruits such as melons, grapes, and berries, and vegetables like cucumber, zucchini, and leafy greens are excellent choices. Avoid spicy, salty, and sour foods, as these can exacerbate Pitta's heat. Hydration is crucial in summer; drink plenty of water, herbal teas, and coconut water to stay cool and refreshed. Physical activity should be moderate and performed during the cooler parts of the day, such as early morning or late evening. Swimming, walking, and gentle yoga can help maintain fitness without overheating the body. Incorporate cooling practices like applying aloe vera gel to the skin and taking cool showers.

Autumn is dominated by the Vata dosha, bringing qualities of dryness, lightness, and variability. The transition from the warmth of summer to the coolness of winter can disrupt Vata, resulting in dry skin, anxiety, and digestive irregularities. To ground and balance Vata, focus on warmth, moisture, and stability in your diet and lifestyle. Opt for warm, cooked foods that are naturally sweet, sour, and salty. Root vegetables, grains, and nourishing oils such as ghee and sesame oil are beneficial. Spices like cinnamon, cardamom, and cumin can aid digestion and provide warmth. Regularity in routine is essential to counteract Vata's erratic nature. Establish a consistent schedule for meals, sleep, and work to provide stability. Self-massage with warm oils like sesame or almond can help moisturize the skin and calm the nervous system. Engage in gentle, grounding exercises like yoga, tai chi, or walking to maintain physical and mental balance.

Winter combines the influences of both Vata and Kapha doshas. Early winter tends to be more Vata-like with its dryness and cold, while late winter takes on Kapha's heavy and damp qualities. To navigate this dual influence, start the winter with Vata-balancing practices and shift to Kapha-balancing strategies as the season progresses. In early winter, maintain a warm, nourishing diet to combat Vata's cold and dry nature. Soups, stews, and casseroles made with root vegetables, grains, and healthy fats are ideal. As winter deepens and Kapha becomes more prominent, gradually incorporate lighter, spicier foods to prevent Kapha buildup. Ginger tea, warm broths, and hearty grains like quinoa and millet are beneficial. Physical activity should be regular and stimulating to counter the lethargy of Kapha and the instability of Vata. Indoor exercises like strength training, brisk walking, and aerobic activities can keep the body warm and energized.

Mindfulness and connection with loved ones are also important in winter to counter the seasonal blues. Engage in hobbies, spend quality time with family and friends, and practice gratitude to bring warmth and joy into your life. By understanding and responding to the seasonal qualities through our diet and lifestyle choices, we can harness the power of Ayurveda to maintain balance and promote overall well-being throughout the year. Embracing these seasonal adjustments allows us to live in harmony with the natural world, embodying the ancient wisdom of Ayurveda in our daily lives.

Staying Balanced Year-Round

Ayurveda, the ancient system of holistic health, emphasizes the importance of aligning our lives with the natural rhythms of the environment. This alignment is particularly crucial when it comes to the changing seasons, each of which has unique characteristics that can influence our physical, mental, and emotional well-being. Understanding how to stay balanced throughout the year by adjusting our diet, lifestyle, and daily routines according to the seasons is a key aspect of Ayurvedic practice. This chapter provides detailed guidance on how to maintain balance year-round, ensuring that we remain healthy and harmonious in every season.

Spring: Renew and Invigorate

Spring is governed by the Kapha dosha, characterized by the qualities of earth and water, making it a time of renewal and growth. As the cold, dry winter transitions into the moist, heavy, and cool spring, there can be an accumulation of Kapha, leading to symptoms such as congestion, sluggishness, and allergies. To counteract these effects, it is essential to adopt practices that invigorate and lighten the body and mind.

Diet plays a crucial role in balancing Kapha during spring. Focus on consuming light, dry, and warm foods. Favor bitter, pungent, and astringent tastes, which help reduce Kapha. Include plenty of fresh greens, sprouts, and spices like ginger, turmeric, and black pepper in your meals. Avoid dairy, heavy oils, and sweet, sour, and salty foods, as they can increase Kapha's heaviness. Incorporate herbal teas, such as dandelion and ginger tea, to aid digestion and detoxification.

Lifestyle adjustments should include regular physical activity to stimulate circulation and dispel Kapha's lethargy. Engage in vigorous exercises like jogging, cycling, or dancing. Start your day with a brisk walk or a dynamic yoga session. Dry brushing and using light, stimulating oils like mustard or sesame for self-massage can further invigorate the system. Spring cleaning, both in your living space and in your diet, can help remove any accumulated toxins and refresh your surroundings.

Summer: Cool and Soothe

Summer, ruled by the Pitta dosha, is characterized by heat, intensity, and brightness. The rising temperatures and longer days can aggravate Pitta, leading to issues like overheating, inflammation, and irritability. To maintain balance during the summer, it is crucial to adopt cooling, soothing, and hydrating practices.

A Pitta-pacifying diet is essential during the summer months. Emphasize foods that are cool, sweet, and mildly astringent. Fresh fruits such as melons, grapes, and berries, along with vegetables like cucumbers, zucchini, and leafy greens, are ideal. Avoid excessively spicy, salty, and sour foods, which can increase internal heat. Incorporate cooling herbs such as mint, coriander, and fennel into your meals. Drinking plenty of water, herbal teas, and coconut water helps stay hydrated and cool.

Physical activities should be performed during the cooler parts of the day, such as early morning or late evening. Opt for moderate exercises like swimming, walking, and gentle yoga to keep the body fit without generating excess heat. Incorporate cooling practices into your daily routine, such as applying aloe vera gel or sandalwood paste to the skin, taking cool showers, and wearing light, breathable clothing made of natural fibers.

Autumn: Ground and Stabilize

Autumn is dominated by the Vata dosha, bringing qualities of dryness, lightness, and variability. The transition from the warmth of summer to the coolness of winter can disrupt Vata, resulting in dry skin, anxiety, and digestive irregularities. To ground and balance Vata during this season, focus on warmth, moisture, and stability in your diet and lifestyle.

A Vata-pacifying diet includes warm, cooked foods that are naturally sweet, sour, and salty. Emphasize root vegetables, grains, and nourishing oils such as ghee and sesame oil. Soups, stews, and casseroles made with warming spices like cinnamon, cardamom, and cloves are beneficial. Avoid cold, raw foods and stimulants like caffeine, which can increase Vata's erratic nature.

Routine and regularity are essential to counteract Vata's variability. Establish consistent daily routines for eating, sleeping, and working to provide stability. Self-massage with warm oils like sesame or almond can help moisturize the skin and calm the nervous system. Engage in gentle, grounding exercises like yoga, tai chi, or walking to maintain physical and mental balance. Practices such as deep breathing, meditation, and spending time in nature can also help stabilize the mind and emotions.

Winter: Warm and Nourish

Winter is a season influenced by both Vata and Kapha doshas. Early winter tends to be more Vata-like with its dryness and cold, while late winter takes on Kapha's heavy and damp qualities. To navigate this dual influence, it is essential to start the winter with Vata-balancing practices and shift to Kapha-balancing strategies as the season progresses.

In early winter, maintain a warm, nourishing diet to combat Vata's cold and dry nature. Soups, stews, and casseroles made with root vegetables, grains, and healthy fats are ideal. Warm drinks like herbal teas and spiced milk can provide comfort and hydration. As winter deepens and Kapha becomes more prominent, gradually incorporate lighter, spicier foods to prevent Kapha buildup. Ginger tea, warm broths, and hearty grains like quinoa and millet are beneficial.

Physical activity should be regular and stimulating to counter the lethargy of Kapha and the instability of Vata. Indoor exercises like strength training, brisk walking, and aerobic activities can keep the body warm and energized. Maintaining a consistent exercise routine is crucial to avoid the sluggishness often associated with winter.

Mindfulness and connection with loved ones are also important in winter to counter the seasonal blues. Engage in hobbies, spend quality time with family and friends, and practice gratitude to bring warmth and joy into your life. Regular self-care routines, such as warm oil massages and relaxing baths, can provide comfort and maintain balance during the colder months.

By understanding the unique qualities of each season and adjusting our diet, lifestyle, and daily routines accordingly, we can stay balanced and healthy throughout the year. Ayurveda offers a comprehensive approach to living in harmony with nature's cycles, ensuring that we remain resilient and vibrant no matter the season. Embracing these seasonal adjustments allows us to embody the wisdom of Ayurveda in our daily lives, promoting overall well-being and harmony with the natural world.

Part 4: Special Topics:

1. Ayurveda for Families

Ayurvedic Practices for Children

Ayurveda, the ancient Indian system of holistic health, provides a comprehensive approach to nurturing the physical, mental, and emotional well-being of individuals of all ages. When it comes to children, Ayurveda offers gentle and effective practices to support their growth and development. These practices not only promote health but also instill a sense of balance and harmony from an early age. This chapter explores various Ayurvedic practices for children, focusing on diet, lifestyle, and natural remedies that can be easily integrated into family routines.

Dietary Guidelines for Children

A balanced diet is fundamental to a child's health and development. In Ayurveda, it is believed that a child's diet should be tailored to their unique constitution (Prakriti) and the changing needs of their growing bodies. Generally, children's diets should be nourishing, easy to digest, and rich in essential nutrients.

Breastfeeding is highly recommended for infants as it provides the ideal nourishment and strengthens the immune system. As children grow, introducing solid foods should be done gradually, starting with easily digestible foods such as rice, lentils, and cooked vegetables. Fresh fruits and vegetables, whole grains, dairy products like milk and ghee, and proteins such as lentils and beans should form the core of a child's diet.

It is essential to incorporate all six tastes (sweet, sour, salty, bitter, pungent, and astringent) in a balanced manner to ensure that all nutritional needs are met. Sweet and nourishing foods like milk, ghee, and grains are particularly beneficial for children as they support growth and provide energy. However, it is important to avoid excessive sugar and processed foods, which can lead to imbalances and health issues.

Herbal teas, such as fennel or chamomile tea, can aid digestion and calm the nervous system. Spices like turmeric, cumin, and ginger, used in moderation, can enhance digestion and boost immunity. Hydration is crucial, so encourage children to drink plenty of water and avoid sugary drinks.

Daily Routines and Lifestyle Practices

Establishing a consistent daily routine (Dinacharya) is crucial for children, as it provides structure and security, which are essential for their development. A regular routine helps regulate bodily functions, supports mental clarity, and promotes emotional stability.

Start the day with a gentle morning routine. Encourage children to wake up early, ideally before sunrise, to align with the natural rhythms of the day. Teach them to begin their day with basic hygiene practices, such as brushing their teeth and washing their face. Tongue scraping, a common Ayurvedic practice, can be introduced as they get older to remove toxins and promote oral health.

A balanced breakfast is important to kickstart the day. Offer warm, nourishing foods such as porridge, oatmeal, or whole-grain toast with ghee. Avoid cold and heavy foods in the morning, as they can dampen digestion.

Physical activity is vital for children's health and development. Encourage outdoor play, yoga, or simple exercises to keep their bodies active and strong. Yoga, in particular, can help improve flexibility, strength, and concentration. Simple poses like the Tree Pose (Vrikshasana) and Cat-Cow Pose (Marjaryasana-Bitilasana) are great for children.

Mental and emotional well-being can be supported through mindfulness and relaxation practices. Teach children simple breathing exercises (Pranayama) to help them manage stress and anxiety. Techniques such as belly breathing or alternate nostril breathing (Nadi Shodhana) are easy for children to learn and can be incorporated into their daily routine.

Bedtime routines should be calming and consistent. Encourage children to go to bed early and at the same time every night. Before bed, activities like reading a book, gentle storytelling, or listening to soothing music can help them unwind. A warm bath with a few drops of lavender oil can promote relaxation and improve sleep quality.

Natural Remedies and Ayurvedic Treatments

Ayurveda offers a variety of natural remedies and treatments that are safe and effective for children. These remedies can address common childhood ailments and support overall health.

For digestive issues, which are common in children, herbs like ginger and fennel can be very beneficial. A mild ginger tea or fennel water can help relieve indigestion and bloating. Hingvastak churna, a blend of digestive herbs, can be sprinkled on food to enhance digestion.

Boosting immunity is crucial for children, especially during the colder months. Chyawanprash, a traditional Ayurvedic herbal jam, is rich in vitamin C and other nutrients that support immune health. Amla (Indian gooseberry), a key ingredient in Chyawanprash, is particularly potent in enhancing immunity and overall vitality.

For respiratory issues like colds and coughs, herbal steam inhalation using eucalyptus or mint can help clear nasal passages and ease breathing. Turmeric milk, known as golden milk, is another excellent remedy. It can be made by adding a teaspoon of turmeric powder to a glass of warm milk, sweetened with a bit of honey.

Skin issues such as rashes or dryness can be addressed with natural oils. Coconut oil or a mixture of turmeric and sandalwood paste can soothe and heal the skin. Regular oil massage (Abhyanga) with warm sesame oil can nourish the skin, improve circulation, and promote overall well-being.

For teething infants, a gentle gum massage with a clean finger dipped in honey can provide relief. Always ensure that the honey is appropriate for the child's age, as it is not recommended for children under one year.

Emotional and Mental Well-Being

Children's emotional and mental well-being is as important as their physical health. Ayurveda emphasizes the need for a loving, supportive environment to nurture a child's emotional health. Spending quality time with family, engaging in creative activities, and fostering open communication are essential.

Teach children the value of mindfulness and gratitude. Simple practices such as keeping a gratitude journal or expressing thankfulness during family meals can instill a positive outlook on life. Encourage them to connect with nature through activities like gardening, nature walks, or simply playing outside, which can have a grounding and calming effect.

Incorporate stories and teachings from Ayurveda that emphasize values like compassion, honesty, and respect for nature. These stories can be a powerful way to impart moral values and life lessons.

By integrating Ayurvedic practices into daily routines, families can support the holistic development of their children. These practices not only promote physical health but also foster mental, emotional, and spiritual well-being. Ayurveda offers a time-tested, natural approach to nurturing children, helping them grow into balanced, healthy, and happy individuals.

Family Meals and Routines

Ayurveda, the ancient science of life and wellness, offers profound wisdom for fostering harmony and health within families. At its core, Ayurveda emphasizes balance, routine, and mindful living, which are particularly beneficial in the context of family meals and daily routines. By integrating Ayurvedic principles into family life, we can create a nurturing environment that supports the physical, emotional, and spiritual well-being of every family member.

Family meals are a cornerstone of Ayurvedic living. In Ayurveda, food is not merely sustenance; it is a powerful tool for maintaining and restoring health. Preparing and sharing meals together strengthens family bonds and ensures that everyone benefits from a balanced diet tailored to their unique constitutions or doshas—Vata, Pitta, and Kapha. Each dosha has specific dietary needs and preferences, and understanding these can help in planning meals that are both nourishing and harmonizing.

For a Vata-dominant family member, who may be prone to dryness, cold, and irregularity, meals should be warm, moist, and grounding. Think of hearty soups, stews, and dishes made with root vegetables, whole grains, and healthy fats. Pitta types, who are naturally fiery and intense, benefit from cooling, calming foods. Fresh fruits, leafy greens, and dairy products like milk and ghee can help balance their heat. Kapha individuals, with their slower metabolism and tendency toward heaviness, thrive on light, stimulating foods. Spices, legumes, and a variety of vegetables can keep their digestive fire strong.

Incorporating these principles into family meals involves creativity and flexibility. For instance, a single meal can be customized to suit different doshas by adjusting spices and side dishes. A simple rice and vegetable dish can be made more grounding with the addition of ghee and warming spices like ginger for Vata, cooling with cilantro and a squeeze of lime for Pitta, and lightened with a touch of black pepper and mustard seeds for Kapha. This way, everyone enjoys the same meal, yet each person receives what they need to stay balanced.

Beyond the specific foods, the manner in which meals are prepared and consumed is crucial in Ayurveda. Cooking is viewed as a sacred act, and the energy and intention of the cook influence the food's vitality. Encourage family members to take turns in meal preparation, infusing their love and care into the process. Eating together, without distractions like television or smartphones, fosters mindful eating and enhances digestion. The atmosphere during meals should be calm and pleasant, with gratitude and appreciation for the food and each other.

Ayurvedic routines extend beyond meals to encompass the entire day. Establishing daily rhythms that align with natural cycles supports overall health and harmony. A consistent routine, or dinacharya, helps regulate the body's internal clock and maintains balance among the doshas. For families, creating a shared daily routine can be both grounding and unifying.

Begin the day early, ideally before sunrise, to harness the freshness and tranquility of the early morning hours. This is a time for self-care practices like brushing teeth, tongue scraping, and oil pulling, which promote oral and overall health. Encourage family members to engage in gentle stretching or yoga to awaken the body and mind, followed by a few minutes of meditation or deep breathing to set a positive tone for the day.

Breakfast should be nourishing and suitable for each dosha. A warm, cooked breakfast like oatmeal or a spiced porridge is generally balancing for all. Lunch, the main meal of the day in Ayurveda, should be hearty and consumed when the digestive fire is strongest, around midday. Dinner should be lighter and eaten early to ensure proper digestion before sleep. Consistency in meal times helps regulate appetite and digestion, contributing to overall well-being.

Incorporate relaxation and bonding time into the evening routine. This can include activities like a family walk, storytelling, or playing a board game. Limiting screen time in the evenings promotes better sleep and more meaningful interactions. Bedtime should be early and consistent, ensuring everyone gets adequate rest to rejuvenate for the next day.

In addition to daily routines, seasonal changes are significant in Ayurveda. Each season brings shifts in doshic balance, and adapting family routines and diets accordingly can prevent imbalances. For example, during the dry, cold months of winter, favoring warm, oily foods and activities that generate internal heat can help balance the Vata dosha, which is predominant in winter. In contrast, the hot, intense summer months call for cooling foods and practices to pacify Pitta.

Family rituals that align with the seasons, such as spring detoxes or autumnal grounding practices, can be deeply bonding and health-enhancing. Simple seasonal activities like gardening in spring, swimming in summer, hiking in autumn, and indoor games in winter can connect the family with nature's rhythms.

Ayurveda also places great importance on emotional well-being. Family support systems play a critical role in managing stress and fostering resilience. Regular family meetings or check-ins can provide a safe space for each member to express their feelings and concerns. Practices like gratitude journaling, where family members share things they are thankful for, can cultivate a positive and supportive family atmosphere.

Ultimately, Ayurveda for families is about creating a balanced, harmonious lifestyle that nurtures each member's body, mind, and spirit. By integrating Ayurvedic principles into family meals and routines, we can foster a healthy, happy family environment that supports lifelong wellness and fulfillment.

Teaching Ayurveda to Kids

Introducing Ayurveda to children is a wonderful way to instill healthy habits and a deep connection to natural living from an early age. Ayurveda, the ancient science of life, provides a holistic approach to health that can be easily adapted to suit the needs and understanding of young minds. By teaching kids about Ayurveda, families can cultivate a sense of balance, mindfulness, and well-being that will benefit them throughout their lives.

Start by introducing the concept of the three doshas—Vata, Pitta, and Kapha—in a way that children can easily grasp. Use simple analogies and relatable examples to explain these fundamental Ayurvedic principles. For instance, you can describe Vata as the energy of movement, like the wind, which can be light and breezy or, when out of balance, like a storm. Pitta can be explained as the energy of transformation, like fire, which is warm and powerful but can also become too hot. Kapha can be likened to the energy of stability, like water and earth, which provides strength and steadiness but can also become heavy and sluggish.

Engage children with interactive and hands-on activities to help them understand their unique constitution and the doshas. Create simple questionnaires or quizzes that they can fill out to discover their predominant dosha. This can be a fun and insightful activity that helps them recognize their own tendencies and traits. Encourage them to observe how they feel at different times of the day, in different seasons, and after eating various foods, helping them to see the practical application of these principles in their daily lives.

Food is a great way to teach kids about Ayurveda. Introduce them to the idea that food is not just for nourishment but also for maintaining balance and health. Involve them in the kitchen and let them participate in preparing meals that are tailored to balance the doshas. Teach them about the tastes (sweet, sour, salty, bitter, pungent, and astringent) and how each taste affects their body and mind. For example, explain that sweet foods can be soothing and grounding, which is beneficial for Vata, while too much sweet can aggravate Kapha. Encourage them to try a variety of foods and recognize how they feel after eating them.

Mindful eating is another crucial aspect of Ayurvedic living that can be taught to kids. Explain the importance of eating slowly, chewing thoroughly, and paying attention to the flavors and textures of their food. Create a calm and pleasant eating environment by turning off screens and sitting together as a family. This not only promotes better digestion but also strengthens family bonds.

Daily routines, or dinacharya, are essential in Ayurveda and can be introduced to children in a fun and engaging way. Establish a consistent routine that includes waking up early, personal hygiene practices, and time for relaxation and play. Teach them about the benefits of waking up with the sun, brushing their teeth, tongue scraping, and oil pulling in the morning. Incorporate simple yoga poses or stretches and a few minutes of meditation or deep breathing into their daily routine to help them start the day with a calm and focused mind.

Sleep is another vital component of health in Ayurveda. Explain the importance of going to bed early and getting enough rest. Create a soothing bedtime routine that includes activities like reading a book, listening to calming music, or practicing gentle stretches to help them wind down. Ensure their sleep environment is comfortable and conducive to restful sleep.

Introduce children to the natural rhythms and cycles of the seasons. Explain how different seasons affect their body and mind and teach them how to adapt their diet and activities accordingly. For example, in the summer, encourage them to eat cooling foods like fruits and vegetables and engage in activities that help them stay cool. In the winter, focus on warming foods and indoor activities that generate heat and energy.

Emotional well-being is a significant aspect of Ayurveda. Teach children about the importance of expressing their emotions and coping with stress. Encourage open communication within the family, allowing them to share their feelings and experiences. Introduce simple practices like journaling, where they can write down their thoughts and feelings, or mindfulness exercises that help them stay present and calm.

Incorporate Ayurvedic herbs and remedies into their daily routine in a safe and age-appropriate manner. Teach them about the benefits of common herbs like turmeric, ginger, and basil, and how they can support their health. Make herbal teas together and explain how these natural remedies can help with digestion, immunity, and overall well-being.

Finally, lead by example. Children learn best by observing the adults around them. Practice Ayurvedic principles in your own life and involve your children in your wellness routines. Show them the joy and benefits of living in harmony with nature and their own unique constitution.

By teaching Ayurveda to kids, you are giving them valuable tools for lifelong health and well-being. This ancient wisdom, adapted to modern living, can help them develop a deep understanding of their own bodies, cultivate healthy habits, and foster a balanced and harmonious life.

2. Ayurveda in the Workplace

Staying Balanced at Work

The modern workplace, with its often hectic pace and high demands, can be a challenging environment to maintain balance and well-being. Ayurveda, the ancient science of life, offers a comprehensive approach to staying balanced at work, enhancing both productivity and personal health. By integrating Ayurvedic principles into daily work routines, individuals can create a harmonious and sustainable approach to professional life.

One of the foundational concepts in Ayurveda is the understanding of the three doshas: Vata, Pitta, and Kapha. Each dosha represents different physiological and psychological characteristics, and recognizing one's predominant dosha can help tailor strategies for maintaining balance at work. For instance, Vata types may struggle with staying grounded and focused, Pitta types might contend with stress and burnout due to their intense nature, and Kapha types could face challenges with motivation and lethargy. By identifying these tendencies, individuals can adopt specific practices to counteract imbalances and enhance their work experience.

Creating a balanced workday begins with a consistent and mindful morning routine. Ayurveda emphasizes the importance of starting the day early, ideally before sunrise, to align with the natural rhythms of the environment. This practice, known as Brahma Muhurta, is considered an auspicious time for activities that foster clarity and vitality. Incorporating morning rituals such as tongue scraping, oil pulling, and gentle yoga or stretching can invigorate the body and mind, setting a positive tone for the day ahead.

Diet plays a crucial role in maintaining balance throughout the workday. Ayurveda recommends consuming the largest meal during midday when the digestive fire, or Agni, is at its strongest. This meal should be nourishing and balanced, incorporating all six tastes (sweet, sour, salty, bitter, pungent, and astringent) to ensure satisfaction and nutritional completeness. Bringing home-cooked meals to work can help avoid the pitfalls of fast food or unhealthy snacks, which can disrupt digestion and energy levels. Including spices like turmeric, cumin, and ginger can aid digestion and enhance mental clarity.

Staying hydrated is essential, but Ayurveda advises sipping warm water or herbal teas rather than cold drinks, which can dampen the digestive fire. Herbal teas such as ginger, mint, or chamomile can be soothing and help maintain focus and calm. Avoiding excessive caffeine is also important, as it can exacerbate Vata imbalances, leading to anxiety and restlessness.

Mindfulness practices are invaluable tools for staying balanced at work. Taking regular breaks to breathe deeply, stretch, or engage in a brief meditation can help reduce stress and maintain mental clarity. The practice of Pranayama, or breath control, can be particularly effective. Simple techniques like Nadi Shodhana (alternate nostril breathing) or Ujjayi (victorious breath) can calm the mind and increase concentration. Setting aside a few minutes every hour to step away from the desk and practice these techniques can make a significant difference in overall well-being.

The physical workspace itself also plays a role in maintaining balance. Ayurveda advocates for a clutter-free, organized environment that promotes positive energy flow. Incorporating elements of nature, such as plants, can enhance the ambiance and provide a calming effect. Ensuring proper lighting, preferably natural light, and good ventilation can improve both mood and productivity. Personalizing the workspace with items that bring joy or inspiration, like family photos or motivational quotes, can also create a more harmonious and supportive environment.

Managing stress is a key aspect of staying balanced at work. Ayurveda offers various strategies to cope with stress, including the use of adaptogenic herbs such as Ashwagandha and Brahmi, which can support the nervous system and enhance resilience. Regular self-massage with warm oil (Abhyanga) can also be deeply relaxing and grounding, helping to counteract the effects of prolonged sitting and mental strain.

Balancing work with regular physical activity is crucial. Incorporating movement into the daily routine, such as walking meetings, taking the stairs, or simple desk exercises, can help counteract the sedentary nature of many jobs. Engaging in a regular exercise regimen outside of work, such as yoga, swimming, or walking in nature, supports overall physical and mental health.

Ayurveda also emphasizes the importance of a balanced work-life dynamic. Setting clear boundaries between work and personal time is essential to prevent burnout and maintain overall well-being. This includes taking time to unplug from digital devices, engaging in hobbies, and spending quality time with loved ones. Practices like spending time in nature, pursuing creative activities, and cultivating a gratitude practice can nourish the soul and provide a counterbalance to the demands of work.

Lastly, fostering positive relationships at work can significantly enhance the work environment. Ayurveda encourages a cooperative and supportive approach to professional interactions. Practicing kindness, active listening, and empathy can create a more harmonious workplace and reduce stress. Regular team-building activities and open communication channels can strengthen connections and improve overall workplace morale.

By integrating these Ayurvedic principles into the workplace, individuals can create a more balanced, productive, and fulfilling professional life. The wisdom of Ayurveda provides practical tools and insights that can help navigate the challenges of modern work, promoting both individual well-being and a healthier work environment. Through mindful practices, proper nutrition, stress management, and a supportive work culture, it is possible to thrive in the workplace while maintaining harmony and balance.

Ayurvedic Tips for Office Life.

Ayurveda, the ancient system of natural healing, offers valuable insights and practices to create balance and well-being in the modern office environment. Office life, with its sedentary nature, constant screen exposure, and high stress levels, can be challenging to one's health. By incorporating Ayurvedic principles, we can cultivate a more harmonious and productive workspace.

Starting the day with a mindful morning routine is essential for setting a positive tone. Ayurveda recommends waking up early, ideally before sunrise, to align with the body's natural rhythms. This quiet time is perfect for self-care practices such as tongue scraping, oil pulling, and gentle yoga or stretching. These activities not only promote physical health but also prepare the mind for the day ahead.

Breakfast should be nourishing yet light, avoiding foods that are too heavy or difficult to digest early in the morning. Warm, cooked meals like oatmeal with spices such as cinnamon and cardamom can provide sustained energy without overwhelming the digestive system. Drinking warm water or herbal tea instead of coffee can also help maintain hydration and gentle stimulation without the jitteriness of caffeine.

When arriving at the office, creating a balanced workspace is key. Ayurveda emphasizes the importance of a clutter-free, organized environment. A tidy desk with minimal distractions can enhance focus and productivity. Incorporating elements of nature, such as plants or a small water fountain, can improve the atmosphere and reduce stress. Natural light is preferable, but if unavailable, ensure good quality lighting to reduce eye strain and fatigue.

Posture and ergonomics play a crucial role in maintaining physical health at work. Sitting for extended periods can lead to various health issues, so it is important to set up the workstation correctly. The chair should support the lower back, feet should rest flat on the floor, and the computer screen should be at eye level to prevent neck strain. Taking regular breaks to stand, stretch, or walk around can alleviate stiffness and improve circulation.

Staying hydrated is vital for maintaining energy and concentration. Ayurveda suggests sipping warm water throughout the day, which is easier on the digestive system than cold water. Herbal teas like ginger, mint, or fennel can provide additional benefits such as improved digestion and mental clarity. It's also important to listen to the body's thirst cues rather than relying solely on scheduled drinking times.

Lunch should be the main meal of the day, eaten when the digestive fire is strongest, typically around midday. Bringing a homemade, balanced meal that includes all six tastes—sweet, sour, salty, bitter, pungent, and astringent—ensures nutritional variety and satisfaction. Avoiding overly processed foods and opting for fresh, whole foods can prevent energy slumps and maintain steady productivity levels. Eating mindfully, away from the desk if possible, allows for better digestion and a mental break from work.

Mindfulness practices can significantly enhance the office experience. Taking a few minutes for deep breathing exercises, such as Pranayama, can reduce stress and clear the mind. Simple techniques like alternate nostril breathing (Nadi Shodhana) or diaphragmatic breathing can be done discreetly at the desk and have immediate calming effects. Incorporating short meditation sessions or even brief walks outdoors during breaks can also rejuvenate the mind and body.

Managing stress is crucial in maintaining overall well-being in the office. Ayurveda offers various strategies to cope with stress effectively. Adaptogenic herbs such as Ashwagandha and Brahmi can support the nervous system and enhance resilience. Aromatherapy, using essential oils like lavender or sandalwood, can create a calming environment and improve mood. Regular self-massage with warm oil (Abhyanga) can also help release tension and promote relaxation.

The afternoon slump is a common challenge in office life. To combat this, Ayurveda suggests light, energizing snacks such as fresh fruit, nuts, or a small portion of dark chocolate. Avoiding heavy, sugary snacks that can lead to a crash later is essential. Gentle stretching or a quick walk can also help re-energize the body and mind during this time.

Balancing work and personal life is another important aspect of Ayurveda. Setting clear boundaries between work and home life can prevent burnout and ensure sufficient rest and rejuvenation. Creating an end-of-day ritual, such as tidying the workspace, reflecting on accomplishments, or practicing gratitude, can provide a sense of closure and transition into personal time.

Evenings should be reserved for relaxation and unwinding. Limiting screen time after work helps improve sleep quality and reduces eye strain. Engaging in calming activities like reading, spending time with loved ones, or pursuing hobbies can create a balanced lifestyle. Ensuring a consistent sleep schedule and creating a restful sleep environment are also vital for maintaining overall health.

By incorporating these Ayurvedic tips into office life, individuals can create a more balanced, healthy, and productive work environment. The principles of Ayurveda offer practical solutions to the challenges of modern office life, fostering well-being and harmony amidst the demands of the workplace. Through mindful practices, proper nutrition, stress management, and creating a supportive work culture, it is possible to thrive in the office while maintaining balance and wellness.

Managing Work Stress

In today's fast-paced world, where stress seems to be an inevitable part of our daily lives, finding ways to manage it effectively has become paramount for maintaining our well-being. The workplace, with its demanding deadlines, high expectations, and constant pressure, can often serve as a breeding ground for stress-related issues. However, Ayurveda, the ancient holistic healing system originating from India, offers invaluable wisdom and practical solutions for managing work stress and promoting balance and harmony in our professional lives.

Ayurveda views the human being as a microcosm of the universe, consisting of the same elemental building blocks found in nature - space, air, fire, water, and earth. According to Ayurvedic principles, when these elements are in balance within the body, mind, and spirit, we experience optimal health and well-being. However, imbalances in these elemental energies can lead to physical and mental disturbances, including stress.

Understanding one's unique constitution, or dosha, is fundamental in Ayurveda for addressing imbalances and promoting harmony. The three doshas - Vata, Pitta, and Kapha - represent different combinations of the five elements and govern various physiological and psychological functions in the body. Each individual has a unique blend of these doshas, which influences their physical characteristics, personality traits, and susceptibility to certain health issues, including stress.

In the context of managing work stress, Ayurveda emphasizes the importance of maintaining balance in all aspects of life, including diet, lifestyle, and daily routines. Here are some key principles and practices from Ayurveda that can help individuals navigate the challenges of the workplace and cultivate resilience in the face of stress:

1. **Mindful Eating**: According to Ayurveda, food is not only nourishment for the body but also for the mind and spirit. Eating mindfully and choosing foods that support your dosha balance can help regulate stress levels. Incorporating nourishing, whole foods such as fresh fruits, vegetables, whole grains, and healthy fats can provide sustained energy and promote mental clarity.
2. **Stress-Reducing Herbs and Supplements**: Ayurveda offers a rich pharmacopeia of herbs and botanicals known for their

adaptogenic and stress-reducing properties. Ashwagandha, Brahmi, Tulsi, and Shatavari are just a few examples of herbs that can help the body adapt to stress, support the nervous system, and promote overall well-being. Consulting with a qualified Ayurvedic practitioner can help determine which herbs are most suitable for individual needs.

3. **Daily Routine (Dinacharya)**: Establishing a daily routine aligned with the natural rhythms of the day is essential for maintaining balance and managing stress. Incorporating practices such as waking up early, practicing yoga or meditation, and setting aside time for self-care activities can help ground and center the mind, allowing for greater resilience in the face of workplace challenges.

4. **Yoga and Pranayama**: The practice of yoga, which includes physical postures (asanas) and breathwork (pranayama), is a powerful tool for reducing stress and promoting relaxation. Incorporating a regular yoga practice into your daily routine can help release tension from the body, calm the mind, and improve overall resilience to stress. Simple pranayama techniques, such as deep belly breathing or alternate nostril breathing, can be practiced discreetly at your desk to alleviate stress in the moment.

5. **Self-awareness and Boundaries**: Cultivating self-awareness and setting healthy boundaries in the workplace are essential for managing stress effectively. Recognizing your own limits, prioritizing tasks, and learning to say no when necessary can help prevent burnout and maintain a sense of balance and well-being.

6. **Mindfulness and Stress Management Techniques**: Incorporating mindfulness practices such as meditation, guided imagery, or progressive muscle relaxation can help reduce stress levels and promote a sense of calm and clarity in the midst of workplace challenges. Taking short breaks throughout the day to practice mindfulness can help reset the nervous system and improve overall resilience to stress.

7. **Work-Life Balance**: Striking a healthy balance between work and personal life is essential for managing stress and promoting overall well-being. Setting boundaries around work hours, unplugging from technology outside of work, and prioritizing time for hobbies, relationships, and self-care activities can help prevent burnout and foster greater satisfaction and fulfillment in both professional and personal domains.

By integrating these Ayurvedic principles and practices into our daily lives, we can cultivate greater resilience, balance, and well-being in the workplace, allowing us to navigate challenges with grace and equanimity. Ayurveda reminds us that true health and happiness are not just the absence of disease or stress but the presence of harmony, balance, and vitality in all aspects of our being.

3. Ayurvedic Travel Tips

Staying Balanced on the Go

Traveling, whether for business or pleasure, can be exhilarating and enriching, offering opportunities for new experiences, cultural exploration, and personal growth. However, the disruptions to routine, changes in environment, and exposure to different foods and climates can also challenge our physical and mental well-being. In the midst of these changes, Ayurveda, the ancient science of life, provides valuable insights and practical tips for staying balanced and healthy while on the go.

Ayurveda teaches us that maintaining balance in our doshas, or unique mind-body constitutions, is key to promoting overall health and well-being. Traveling can disrupt this balance, leading to symptoms such as digestive disturbances, fatigue, anxiety, and insomnia. By incorporating Ayurvedic principles into our travel routines, we can support our dosha balance and mitigate the effects of travel stressors. Here are some Ayurvedic travel tips to help you stay balanced on the go:

1. **Prepare Mindfully**: Before embarking on your journey, take time to prepare mindfully. Pack thoughtfully, considering the climate and activities at your destination, as well as any special dietary or medical needs. Plan your itinerary with attention to pacing and downtime to prevent exhaustion and overwhelm.
2. **Stay Hydrated**: Traveling can dehydrate the body, especially if you're flying or visiting warmer climates. Drink plenty of water throughout your journey to stay hydrated and support digestion, elimination, and overall vitality. Opt for room-temperature or warm water, as cold beverages can dampen digestive fire (agni).
3. **Eat Mindfully**: While exploring new cuisines is one of the joys of travel, be mindful of your dietary choices to support your dosha balance. Stick to freshly prepared, whole foods whenever possible, and avoid heavy, processed, or excessively spicy foods that may aggravate digestion. If dining out, consider ordering dishes that are familiar and easy to digest, such as steamed vegetables, soups, or grains.
4. **Maintain Daily Routines**: Traveling can disrupt our usual routines, but maintaining consistency in daily habits can help anchor us amidst change. Try to wake up and go to bed at the

same time each day, even if it means adjusting to a new time zone. Incorporate daily self-care practices such as meditation, yoga, or gentle exercise to ground and center yourself.
5. **Support Digestion**: Digestive disturbances are common during travel due to changes in diet, schedule, and environment. To support healthy digestion, consider taking digestive herbs or supplements such as triphala or ginger before meals. Sip on warm herbal teas like ginger, fennel, or peppermint to aid digestion and soothe any discomfort.
6. **Stay Active**: Traveling often involves long periods of sitting or standing, which can lead to stiffness and fatigue. Stay active during your journey by stretching, walking, or practicing yoga whenever possible. Incorporating movement into your travel routine can help improve circulation, relieve tension, and boost energy levels.
7. **Rest and Recharge**: Traveling can be physically and mentally demanding, so it's essential to prioritize rest and relaxation. Listen to your body's cues and take breaks when needed. Practice deep breathing or relaxation techniques to calm the mind and promote restful sleep, especially if you're dealing with jet lag or insomnia.
8. **Stay Grounded**: Amidst the whirlwind of travel, it's easy to feel unmoored and disconnected from our roots. Take time to connect with nature, whether it's a walk in the park, a swim in the ocean, or simply pausing to admire the beauty of your surroundings. Grounding practices such as walking barefoot on grass or sand can help restore balance and vitality.

By incorporating these Ayurvedic travel tips into your journey, you can support your dosha balance, enhance your travel experience, and return home feeling rejuvenated and refreshed. Remember that travel is not just about reaching your destination but also about the journey itself, and embracing the wisdom of Ayurveda can help you navigate that journey with grace and ease.

Travel-Friendly Ayurvedic Practices

Traveling has always been an integral part of human experience, offering opportunities for exploration, adventure, and personal growth. Whether you're embarking on a business trip, a family vacation, or a solo adventure, traveling can be both exhilarating and challenging, especially when it comes to maintaining balance and well-being amidst the disruptions of routine, changes in environment, and exposure to new experiences.

In the ancient science of Ayurveda, which originated in India over 5,000 years ago, maintaining balance in mind, body, and spirit is considered essential for promoting optimal health and well-being. Ayurveda offers a treasure trove of practical wisdom and time-tested practices that are perfectly suited for travelers seeking to stay healthy, grounded, and balanced on the go. These travel-friendly Ayurvedic practices can help you navigate the challenges of travel with grace and ease:

1. **Mindful Eating**: One of the joys of travel is experiencing new cuisines and flavors from around the world. However, eating mindfully is key to supporting digestion and maintaining balance while on the go. Choose fresh, whole foods whenever possible, and avoid heavy, processed, or excessively spicy foods that may disrupt digestion. Opt for simple, nourishing meals that are easy to digest, such as soups, steamed vegetables, and grains. Pack healthy snacks like nuts, seeds, and fruits to tide you over between meals and prevent energy crashes.
2. **Hydration**: Traveling can dehydrate the body, especially if you're flying or visiting warmer climates. Stay hydrated by drinking plenty of water throughout your journey. Opt for room-temperature or warm water, as cold beverages can dampen digestive fire (agni). Herbal teas like ginger, fennel, or peppermint can also help support digestion and hydration while on the go.
3. **Herbal Supplements**: Ayurveda offers a rich pharmacopeia of herbs and botanicals known for their adaptogenic and immune-supporting properties. Consider taking travel-friendly herbal supplements such as triphala, ashwagandha, or amla to support digestion, boost immunity, and promote overall well-being while

traveling. Consult with a qualified Ayurvedic practitioner to determine which herbs are most suitable for your individual needs.
4. **Daily Routines**: Traveling can disrupt our usual routines, but maintaining consistency in daily habits is essential for staying grounded and balanced on the go. Incorporate Ayurvedic self-care practices into your travel routine, such as meditation, yoga, or gentle exercise, to help center and calm the mind amidst the whirlwind of travel. Establishing a daily routine aligned with the natural rhythms of the day can help anchor you amidst change and promote a sense of stability and well-being.
5. **Breathing Exercises**: Deep breathing exercises, or pranayama, are powerful tools for reducing stress and promoting relaxation while traveling. Practice simple pranayama techniques such as deep belly breathing, alternate nostril breathing, or the 4-7-8 breath to calm the mind, soothe the nervous system, and enhance overall resilience to travel stressors. These techniques can be practiced discreetly anytime, anywhere, making them perfect for travelers on the go.
6. **Aromatherapy**: Aromatherapy, or the use of essential oils, is another travel-friendly Ayurvedic practice that can help promote balance and well-being while on the go. Pack travel-sized bottles of calming essential oils such as lavender, chamomile, or sandalwood to use during your journey. Inhaling these soothing scents can help alleviate travel-related stress and anxiety, promote relaxation, and enhance overall travel experience.
7. **Mindfulness**: Traveling offers countless opportunities for sensory stimulation and cultural immersion, but it can also be overwhelming at times. Practice mindfulness during your travels by staying present and engaged with your surroundings. Take time to savor the sights, sounds, and smells of your destination, and cultivate gratitude for the experiences and connections you encounter along the way. Mindfulness can help reduce stress, enhance appreciation, and enrich your travel experience with a sense of presence and purpose.
8. **Rest and Rejuvenation**: Traveling can be physically and mentally demanding, so it's essential to prioritize rest and rejuvenation during your journey. Listen to your body's cues and take breaks when needed. Allow yourself time to rest, recharge, and integrate your experiences. Practice deep relaxation techniques such as yoga nidra, progressive muscle relaxation, or

guided imagery to promote restful sleep and rejuvenate the body and mind after a long day of travel.

By incorporating these travel-friendly Ayurvedic practices into your journey, you can support your overall well-being, enhance your travel experience, and return home feeling refreshed, rejuvenated, and ready to take on the world. Remember that travel is not just about reaching your destination but also about the journey itself, and embracing the wisdom of Ayurveda can help you navigate that journey with grace, ease, and joy.

Adapting Your Routine

Traveling, whether for business or pleasure, presents a unique set of challenges and opportunities for maintaining balance and well-being. The disruptions to routine, changes in environment, and exposure to new experiences can impact our physical, mental, and emotional health. In the ancient science of Ayurveda, which originated in India over 5,000 years ago, maintaining balance in mind, body, and spirit is considered essential for promoting optimal health and well-being. Ayurveda offers invaluable wisdom and practical tips for adapting your routine to support your well-being while traveling.

1. **Dosha Balancing**: Ayurveda teaches us that each individual has a unique mind-body constitution, or dosha, which influences our physical characteristics, personality traits, and susceptibility to imbalances. Vata, Pitta, and Kapha are the three doshas, representing different combinations of the five elements - space, air, fire, water, and earth. Understanding your dominant dosha and how it may be affected by travel can help you adapt your routine to maintain balance and well-being.
    - Vata individuals tend to be creative, energetic, and prone to anxiety and digestive disturbances when out of balance. Travel can exacerbate Vata imbalances due to its unpredictable nature and changes in routine. Vata individuals should prioritize grounding practices such as meditation, warm nourishing foods, and regular meal times to stay grounded and centered while traveling.
    - Pitta individuals are ambitious, driven, and prone to stress and irritability when out of balance. Travel can aggravate Pitta imbalances due to the demands of schedules and

deadlines. Pitta individuals should prioritize cooling and calming practices such as meditation, gentle exercise, and avoiding excessive heat and spicy foods to stay balanced and relaxed while traveling.
    - Kapha individuals are steady, nurturing, and prone to lethargy and congestion when out of balance. Travel can exacerbate Kapha imbalances due to its sedentary nature and exposure to new environments. Kapha individuals should prioritize invigorating practices such as vigorous exercise, stimulating foods and herbs, and maintaining a sense of adventure to stay energized and vibrant while traveling.
2. **Maintaining Consistency**: While traveling often involves disruptions to routine, maintaining consistency in daily habits is essential for supporting balance and well-being. Even if your schedule varies from day to day, aim to wake up and go to bed at the same time each day to regulate your body's internal clock. Incorporate Ayurvedic self-care practices such as meditation, yoga, or gentle exercise into your daily routine to help ground and center yourself amidst the whirlwind of travel.
3. **Mindful Eating**: Eating mindfully is key to supporting digestion and maintaining balance while traveling. While exploring new cuisines and flavors is one of the joys of travel, be mindful of your dietary choices to support your dosha balance. Choose fresh, whole foods whenever possible, and avoid heavy, processed, or excessively spicy foods that may disrupt digestion. Pack healthy snacks like nuts, seeds, and fruits to tide you over between meals and prevent energy crashes.
4. **Hydration**: Traveling can dehydrate the body, especially if you're flying or visiting warmer climates. Stay hydrated by drinking plenty of water throughout your journey. Opt for room-temperature or warm water, as cold beverages can dampen digestive fire (agni). Herbal teas like ginger, fennel, or peppermint can also help support digestion and hydration while on the go.
5. **Rest and Rejuvenation**: Traveling can be physically and mentally demanding, so it's essential to prioritize rest and rejuvenation during your journey. Listen to your body's cues and take breaks when needed. Allow yourself time to rest, recharge, and integrate your experiences. Practice deep relaxation techniques such as yoga nidra, progressive muscle relaxation, or

guided imagery to promote restful sleep and rejuvenate the body and mind after a long day of travel.
6. **Flexibility and Adaptability**: Above all, remember to approach travel with a spirit of flexibility and adaptability. Embrace the unexpected and be open to new experiences and opportunities for growth. Allow yourself to go with the flow and adjust your plans as needed to accommodate changes in schedule, environment, and circumstances. By cultivating a mindset of openness and resilience, you can navigate the challenges of travel with grace, ease, and joy.

By incorporating these Ayurvedic travel tips into your journey, you can adapt your routine to support your well-being, enhance your travel experience, and return home feeling refreshed, rejuvenated, and ready to take on the world. Remember that travel is not just about reaching your destination but also about the journey itself, and embracing the wisdom of Ayurveda can help you navigate that journey with grace, ease, and vitality.

Part 5: Deepening Your Practice

1. Advanced Ayurvedic Techniques

Rasayana (Rejuvenation Therapy)

In the vast and ancient tradition of Ayurveda, there exists a profound branch dedicated to the art and science of rejuvenation known as Rasayana. Rooted in the Sanskrit word "rasa," meaning essence or juice, Rasayana therapies aim to enhance vitality, promote longevity, and restore balance to the body, mind, and spirit. As one of the most advanced and sophisticated practices within Ayurveda, Rasayana encompasses a holistic approach to well-being that integrates dietary guidelines, herbal formulations, lifestyle recommendations, and spiritual practices to rejuvenate and nourish the entire being.

1. **The Philosophy of Rasayana**: At its core, Rasayana embodies the timeless Ayurvedic principle of preserving and promoting health before the onset of disease. Rather than simply treating symptoms, Rasayana seeks to address the root causes of imbalance and restore the body's innate intelligence and vitality. Drawing upon the wisdom of ancient texts such as the Charaka Samhita and the Sushruta Samhita, Rasayana emphasizes the importance of holistic health, longevity, and spiritual evolution as interconnected aspects of well-being.
2. **Types of Rasayana**: Rasayana therapies are classified into two main categories: Kutipraveshika Rasayana and Achara Rasayana. Kutipraveshika Rasayana involves a more intensive and structured approach to rejuvenation, often requiring a period of seclusion, specialized diet, and herbal supplementation under the guidance of a qualified Ayurvedic practitioner. Achara Rasayana, on the other hand, focuses on incorporating lifestyle practices and dietary habits that promote longevity and vitality in daily life.
3. **Benefits of Rasayana**: The benefits of Rasayana therapy are manifold and encompass physical, mental, and emotional well-being. From strengthening the immune system and improving digestion to enhancing cognitive function and promoting emotional resilience, Rasayana therapies are renowned for their ability to nourish and rejuvenate every aspect of the individual. By supporting cellular regeneration, optimizing metabolic function,

and balancing the doshas, Rasayana fosters a state of vibrant health, vitality, and longevity.
4. **Rasayana Diet and Nutrition**: Central to Rasayana therapy is the concept of Ahara Rasayana, or rejuvenating diet. Ahara Rasayana emphasizes the consumption of nutrient-dense foods that are easily digestible, nourishing, and balancing to the doshas. Fresh fruits, vegetables, whole grains, legumes, nuts, seeds, and healthy fats are staples of the Rasayana diet, while processed foods, refined sugars, and artificial additives are minimized or avoided altogether. Herbal formulations such as Chyawanprash, Brahma Rasayana, and Amalaki Rasayana are also commonly used to support cellular rejuvenation and enhance vitality.
5. **Rasayana Lifestyle Practices**: In addition to dietary guidelines, Rasayana encompasses a variety of lifestyle practices that promote longevity and well-being. Daily routines (Dinacharya), seasonal routines (Ritucharya), and spiritual practices (Sadhana) are integral aspects of Rasayana therapy. Regular exercise, adequate rest, stress management techniques, and mind-body practices such as yoga, meditation, and pranayama are encouraged to support overall health and vitality.
6. **Personalized Rasayana Protocols**: Rasayana therapies are highly individualized, taking into account each person's unique constitution, imbalances, and health goals. A qualified Ayurvedic practitioner will conduct a thorough assessment of the individual's physical, mental, and emotional health before designing a personalized Rasayana protocol tailored to their specific needs. This may include dietary modifications, herbal supplementation, lifestyle recommendations, and spiritual practices tailored to support rejuvenation and well-being.
7. **Integrating Rasayana into Modern Life**: While Rasayana therapies have been practiced for thousands of years, they remain relevant and applicable in the modern world. By integrating Rasayana principles into our daily lives, we can cultivate greater health, vitality, and resilience in the face of stress, pollution, and other modern-day challenges. Whether through mindful eating, regular exercise, stress management techniques, or spiritual practices, Rasayana offers a roadmap to vibrant health and longevity that is accessible to everyone.

In conclusion, Rasayana represents a pinnacle of Ayurvedic wisdom and expertise, offering a comprehensive approach to rejuvenation and well-being that encompasses every aspect of the individual - body, mind, and spirit. By embracing the principles and practices of Rasayana, we can unlock the secrets to longevity, vitality, and radiant health, and cultivate a life of true well-being and fulfillment.

Advanced Herbal Treatments

Within the rich tapestry of Ayurvedic healing modalities, herbal treatments stand as pillars of therapeutic efficacy and profound wisdom. For millennia, Ayurvedic practitioners have harnessed the healing power of herbs to address a wide range of health concerns, from simple ailments to chronic diseases. Advanced herbal treatments represent a sophisticated and nuanced approach to healing, drawing upon the intricate knowledge of botanical medicine passed down through generations of Ayurvedic scholars and practitioners.

1. **The Science of Herbal Medicine**: At the heart of Ayurvedic herbal treatments lies a deep understanding of the medicinal properties of plants and their effects on the body, mind, and spirit. Each herb is thought to possess a unique combination of tastes, energies, and actions that can be harnessed to restore balance and promote health. Through the principles of Rasa (taste), Virya (potency), and Vipaka (post-digestive effect), Ayurvedic practitioners tailor herbal formulations to address the specific imbalances and constitution of each individual.
2. **Herbal Formulations**: Ayurvedic herbal treatments often take the form of complex formulations known as Rasayanas, Arishtas, Asavas, Churnas, Ghritas, and Kwathas, among others. These formulations may contain a blend of herbs, minerals, metals, and other natural ingredients carefully selected and combined to enhance their therapeutic efficacy and bioavailability. Depending on the nature of the ailment and the needs of the individual, herbal formulations may be administered orally, topically, or as part of specialized therapies such as Panchakarma.
3. **Classical Texts and Traditions**: The knowledge of herbal medicine in Ayurveda is preserved and transmitted through classical texts such as the Charaka Samhita, Sushruta Samhita, and Astanga Hridaya, as well as through oral traditions passed down

from teacher to student. These texts provide detailed descriptions of hundreds of herbs, their properties, indications, contraindications, and methods of preparation. By adhering to the principles outlined in these ancient texts, Ayurvedic practitioners ensure the integrity and efficacy of their herbal treatments.
4. **Indications and Contraindications**: Advanced herbal treatments in Ayurveda are tailored to address the specific needs and imbalances of each individual. Before prescribing an herbal formulation, a qualified Ayurvedic practitioner conducts a thorough assessment of the patient's constitution, doshic imbalances, current health status, and any underlying conditions. Based on this assessment, the practitioner selects herbs and formulations that are most appropriate for the individual, taking into account factors such as taste, potency, post-digestive effect, and potential interactions with other medications.
5. **Therapeutic Efficacy**: Ayurvedic herbal treatments are renowned for their therapeutic efficacy in addressing a wide range of health concerns. From common ailments such as digestive disorders, respiratory infections, and skin conditions to chronic diseases such as arthritis, diabetes, and autoimmune disorders, herbal treatments offer safe, effective, and sustainable solutions for promoting health and well-being. By addressing the root causes of illness and restoring balance to the body, mind, and spirit, Ayurvedic herbal treatments support the body's innate healing capacity and facilitate long-term wellness.
6. **Integration with Modern Medicine**: While Ayurvedic herbal treatments have been practiced for thousands of years, they continue to evolve and adapt to the changing needs of modern society. Today, Ayurvedic herbs and formulations are increasingly being studied and validated through scientific research, providing evidence for their efficacy and safety. Many modern practitioners of integrative medicine incorporate Ayurvedic herbal treatments into their practice, recognizing the complementary nature of Ayurveda and modern biomedicine in promoting holistic health and wellness.
7. **Accessibility and Sustainability**: One of the greatest strengths of Ayurvedic herbal treatments lies in their accessibility and sustainability. Unlike synthetic drugs, which often come with a host of side effects and environmental concerns, Ayurvedic herbs are natural, renewable resources that are cultivated, harvested, and

processed with care and respect for the earth. By supporting local farmers and sustainable practices, Ayurvedic herbal treatments contribute to the health of individuals, communities, and the planet as a whole.

In conclusion, advanced herbal treatments represent a cornerstone of Ayurvedic healing, offering safe, effective, and sustainable solutions for promoting health and well-being. Rooted in ancient wisdom and guided by modern science, Ayurvedic herbal treatments continue to provide a beacon of hope and healing in an increasingly complex world. By harnessing the healing power of nature and honoring the wisdom of the ages, we can cultivate a life of vitality, resilience, and radiant health.

Deeper Detox Practices

In the quest for optimal health and vitality, detoxification holds a central place in Ayurvedic healing practices. While many people are familiar with basic detox methods such as dietary cleanses and herbal teas, Ayurveda offers deeper detox practices that target the root causes of imbalance and toxicity in the body, mind, and spirit. These advanced detox techniques draw upon the ancient wisdom of Ayurveda to purify the body's tissues, eliminate accumulated toxins, and rejuvenate the entire being.

1. **Understanding Detoxification in Ayurveda**: In Ayurveda, detoxification is viewed as a holistic process that encompasses not only the physical body but also the mind and emotions. According to Ayurvedic principles, toxins, or "ama," accumulate in the body as a result of poor digestion, improper lifestyle habits, environmental pollutants, and emotional stress. These toxins can disrupt the body's natural functions, leading to a wide range of health issues. Detoxification in Ayurveda aims to remove ama from the body and restore balance to the doshas, or mind-body constitutions.
2. **Panchakarma Therapy**: Panchakarma is perhaps the most renowned and comprehensive detoxification therapy in Ayurveda. Derived from the Sanskrit words "pancha" meaning five and "karma" meaning action, Panchakarma involves a series of specialized treatments that target different organs and systems of the body to eliminate toxins and restore balance. These treatments include:

- **Abhyanga (Oil Massage)**: Warm herbal oils are applied to the body in a rhythmic fashion to loosen toxins, improve circulation, and nourish the tissues.
- **Swedana (Steam Therapy)**: The body is subjected to steam therapy to induce sweating and further eliminate toxins through the skin.
- **Vamana (Therapeutic Vomiting)**: Controlled vomiting is induced to expel excess mucus and toxins from the upper respiratory tract and stomach.
- **Virechana (Purgation Therapy)**: Herbal laxatives are administered to promote bowel movements and cleanse the intestines of accumulated toxins.
- **Basti (Enema Therapy)**: Medicated enemas are used to cleanse the colon and remove toxins from the lower digestive tract.
- **Nasya (Nasal Therapy)**: Herbal oils or powders are administered through the nasal passages to cleanse the sinuses and promote respiratory health.

Panchakarma therapy is typically conducted under the guidance of a qualified Ayurvedic practitioner and tailored to the individual's constitution, health status, and specific detoxification needs.

3. **Shirodhara Therapy**: Shirodhara is a deeply relaxing and rejuvenating therapy that involves the continuous pouring of warm herbal oil or medicated liquids over the forehead. This gentle stream of oil stimulates the third eye (Ajna) chakra and induces a state of deep relaxation, promoting mental clarity, emotional balance, and stress relief. Shirodhara is often used as a complementary therapy to Panchakarma or as a standalone treatment for detoxification and rejuvenation of the nervous system.
4. **Herbal Detoxification Formulas**: Ayurveda offers a wide range of herbal formulations known as "kashayas," "arishtas," "asavas," and "choornas" that are specifically designed to support detoxification and elimination of toxins from the body. These formulations typically contain a blend of herbs, spices, and natural ingredients with purifying, cleansing, and rejuvenating properties. Common detoxifying herbs used in Ayurveda include triphala, neem, turmeric, ginger, and guggulu, among others. These herbal

formulas can be taken orally as teas, decoctions, powders, or tablets to support the body's natural detoxification processes.
5. **Dietary Cleansing**: In addition to specialized therapies, Ayurveda emphasizes the importance of dietary cleansing as a fundamental aspect of detoxification. Fasting, mono-dieting, and seasonal cleanses are common dietary practices used in Ayurveda to support digestion, eliminate toxins, and rejuvenate the body. During a cleanse, individuals may consume light, easily digestible foods such as kitchari (a simple rice and lentil dish), vegetable soups, steamed vegetables, and herbal teas. By simplifying the diet and avoiding heavy, processed, and allergenic foods, the digestive system is given a chance to rest and reset, allowing toxins to be eliminated more effectively.
6. **Mind-Body Detox Practices**: Detoxification in Ayurveda extends beyond the physical body to encompass the mind and emotions as well. Stress, negative emotions, and mental toxins can accumulate in the mind and disrupt overall well-being. Mind-body practices such as meditation, pranayama (breathwork), yoga, and mindfulness are powerful tools for detoxifying the mind and promoting emotional balance. By cultivating awareness, presence, and inner peace, these practices help to release stored emotions, clear mental clutter, and promote mental clarity and emotional resilience.
7. **Integration with Lifestyle Practices**: Sustainable detoxification in Ayurveda is not a one-time event but rather a lifestyle approach that integrates daily habits and practices to support ongoing detoxification and rejuvenation. Ayurvedic lifestyle practices such as Dinacharya (daily routine), Ritucharya (seasonal routine), and Sadvritta (ethical living) play a crucial role in maintaining balance and preventing the accumulation of toxins in the body and mind. By incorporating practices such as regular exercise, adequate sleep, stress management, and mindful eating into daily life, individuals can support their body's natural detoxification processes and promote long-term health and vitality.

In conclusion, advanced detox practices in Ayurveda offer a comprehensive and holistic approach to cleansing and rejuvenating the body, mind, and spirit. By incorporating specialized therapies, herbal formulations, dietary cleansing, mind-body practices, and lifestyle adjustments, individuals can support their body's natural detoxification processes and unlock the keys to vibrant health, vitality, and longevity. Whether as a standalone therapy or as part of a broader wellness regimen, advanced detox practices in Ayurveda provide a roadmap to optimal health and well-being in today's modern world.

2. Integrating Ayurveda with Other Practices

Combining Ayurveda with Modern Medicine

In the ever-evolving landscape of healthcare, the integration of traditional and modern healing modalities has emerged as a powerful paradigm for promoting holistic health and well-being. At the intersection of ancient wisdom and cutting-edge science lies a profound opportunity for collaboration and synergy between Ayurveda, the ancient healing system of India, and modern medicine. By integrating the strengths of both systems, individuals can access a comprehensive approach to health that addresses the root causes of illness and promotes optimal wellness on all levels - physical, mental, and emotional.

1. **Understanding Ayurveda and Modern Medicine**: Ayurveda and modern medicine represent two distinct yet complementary approaches to healing. While Ayurveda is rooted in the ancient wisdom of India and emphasizes a holistic understanding of health based on the principles of balance and harmony, modern medicine is grounded in empirical research and scientific methodology, focusing on the diagnosis and treatment of specific diseases using pharmaceuticals and surgical interventions. By understanding the strengths and limitations of each system, individuals can leverage the best of both worlds to optimize their health outcomes.
2. **Complementary Approaches to Healing**: Ayurveda and modern medicine offer complementary approaches to healing that address different aspects of the individual's health and well-being. While modern medicine excels in acute care, emergency medicine, and the management of complex diseases, Ayurveda shines in preventive healthcare, chronic disease management, and promoting overall vitality and resilience. By integrating Ayurvedic principles such as diet, lifestyle, and herbal medicine with modern medical interventions, individuals can enhance the effectiveness of their treatment plans and support their body's innate healing capacity.
3. **Personalized Healthcare**: One of the key strengths of Ayurveda is its emphasis on personalized healthcare tailored to the unique constitution, imbalances, and needs of each individual. Ayurvedic practitioners conduct a thorough assessment of the patient's physical, mental, and emotional health using techniques

such as pulse diagnosis (Nadi Pariksha) and tongue examination (Jivha Pariksha) to identify imbalances and develop personalized treatment plans. By integrating Ayurvedic diagnostics with modern medical tests and assessments, healthcare providers can gain a more comprehensive understanding of the individual's health status and tailor treatment strategies accordingly.

4. **Lifestyle Medicine**: Ayurveda places great emphasis on lifestyle factors such as diet, exercise, sleep, stress management, and daily routines as key determinants of health and well-being. These lifestyle factors play a crucial role in preventing disease, optimizing health, and promoting longevity. By incorporating Ayurvedic lifestyle recommendations into their daily routines, individuals can support their body's natural healing processes, reduce the risk of chronic disease, and enhance their overall quality of life. Lifestyle medicine complements modern medical interventions by addressing underlying lifestyle factors that contribute to disease and promoting long-term wellness.

5. **Herbal Medicine and Nutritional Supplements**: Ayurveda offers a rich pharmacopeia of herbs, botanicals, and nutritional supplements that have been used for millennia to promote health and treat a wide range of ailments. Many of these herbs and supplements have been studied and validated through modern scientific research, providing evidence for their efficacy and safety. By integrating Ayurvedic herbs and nutritional supplements into their treatment plans, individuals can enhance the effectiveness of modern medical interventions, reduce side effects, and support their body's natural healing processes. From adaptogenic herbs that support stress resilience to digestive herbs that promote gut health, Ayurvedic botanicals offer a wealth of therapeutic benefits that can complement modern medical treatments.

6. **Mind-Body Medicine**: Ayurveda recognizes the intimate connection between the mind and body and emphasizes the importance of mental and emotional well-being in promoting overall health. Mind-body practices such as yoga, meditation, pranayama (breathwork), and mindfulness are integral aspects of Ayurvedic healing that promote relaxation, stress reduction, and emotional balance. These practices have been shown to have profound effects on the nervous system, immune system, and hormonal balance, supporting overall health and resilience. By integrating mind-body practices into their healthcare routine,

individuals can enhance the effectiveness of modern medical treatments and cultivate greater harmony and balance in their lives.
7. **Collaborative Care Teams**: Integrating Ayurveda with modern medicine requires collaboration and communication between healthcare providers from different disciplines. Collaborative care teams that include Ayurvedic practitioners, allopathic physicians, nurses, dietitians, and other healthcare professionals can provide comprehensive, patient-centered care that addresses the unique needs and preferences of each individual. By working together, healthcare providers can leverage the strengths of each system, share knowledge and expertise, and develop integrated treatment plans that optimize health outcomes and promote holistic well-being.

In conclusion, integrating Ayurveda with modern medicine offers a powerful approach to health and healing that combines the strengths of both systems to promote holistic well-being. By leveraging the personalized, preventive, and lifestyle-focused approach of Ayurveda with the diagnostic and therapeutic advancements of modern medicine, individuals can access a comprehensive healthcare model that addresses the root causes of illness and supports optimal health on all levels - physical, mental, and emotional. Through collaboration, communication, and shared decision-making, healthcare providers can work together to deliver patient-centered care that honors the wisdom of ancient traditions while embracing the innovations of modern science.

Integrating Other Holistic Practices

In the pursuit of holistic health and well-being, Ayurveda embraces the integration of various holistic practices from around the world. By combining the ancient wisdom of Ayurveda with other complementary healing modalities, individuals can access a diverse toolkit of approaches to support their journey towards optimal health on all levels - physical, mental, emotional, and spiritual. Integrating other holistic practices with Ayurveda offers a comprehensive and personalized approach to healing that honors the uniqueness of each individual and addresses the interconnectedness of mind, body, and spirit.

1. **Traditional Chinese Medicine (TCM)**: Like Ayurveda, Traditional Chinese Medicine (TCM) is a holistic healing system that has been practiced for thousands of years. TCM encompasses a range of modalities including acupuncture, herbal medicine, dietary therapy, qigong, and tai chi, all of which aim to restore balance and harmony to the body's energy systems. Integrating TCM with Ayurveda allows individuals to access a broader range of healing tools and perspectives, enhancing the effectiveness of their treatment plans and promoting overall well-being.
2. **Yoga and Meditation**: Yoga and meditation are integral aspects of Ayurvedic healing that promote physical, mental, and emotional balance. Yoga combines physical postures (asanas), breathwork (pranayama), and meditation to cultivate strength, flexibility, and inner peace. Meditation practices such as mindfulness meditation, loving-kindness meditation, and transcendental meditation promote relaxation, stress reduction, and emotional resilience. Integrating yoga and meditation with Ayurveda allows individuals to cultivate a deeper connection to themselves and support their body's natural healing processes.
3. **Massage Therapy**: Massage therapy is a powerful healing modality that has been used for centuries to promote relaxation, relieve tension, and enhance overall well-being. Ayurvedic massage techniques such as Abhyanga (oil massage) and Shirodhara (oil pouring) are deeply nourishing and rejuvenating, promoting circulation, lymphatic drainage, and detoxification. Integrating massage therapy with Ayurveda allows individuals to experience

profound relaxation and rejuvenation while supporting their body's natural healing processes.

4. **Energy Healing**: Energy healing modalities such as Reiki, pranic healing, and acupuncture focus on balancing the body's energy systems to promote health and well-being. These practices work on the subtle energy body to remove blockages, restore flow, and promote healing on all levels - physical, mental, emotional, and spiritual. Integrating energy healing with Ayurveda allows individuals to address imbalances in their energy systems and promote overall harmony and vitality.

5. **Nutritional Therapy**: Nutrition plays a crucial role in Ayurvedic healing, with diet considered one of the pillars of health. Ayurvedic dietary guidelines emphasize whole, seasonal, and locally sourced foods that are nourishing and balancing to each individual's constitution. Integrating nutritional therapy with Ayurveda allows individuals to optimize their diet to support their unique health needs and goals, promoting digestive health, immunity, and overall vitality.

6. **Herbal Medicine**: Herbal medicine is a cornerstone of Ayurvedic healing that harnesses the healing power of plants to promote health and well-being. Ayurvedic herbs such as ashwagandha, turmeric, and triphala have been used for centuries to support various aspects of health, from stress reduction and immune support to digestive health and detoxification. Integrating herbal medicine with Ayurveda allows individuals to access a wide range of botanical remedies to support their body's natural healing processes.

7. **Mind-Body Practices**: Mind-body practices such as breathwork, visualization, and somatic experiencing promote awareness, relaxation, and emotional resilience. These practices work on the interconnectedness of mind and body to promote healing and well-being. Integrating mind-body practices with Ayurveda allows individuals to cultivate greater awareness of their thoughts, emotions, and sensations, supporting their journey towards holistic health and wellness.

8. **Spiritual Practices**: Spiritual practices such as prayer, gratitude, and connection to nature are integral aspects of Ayurvedic healing that promote a sense of connection, purpose, and meaning in life. These practices nourish the soul and support overall well-being. Integrating spiritual practices with Ayurveda allows individuals to

cultivate a deeper connection to themselves and the world around them, fostering a sense of wholeness and harmony.

In conclusion, integrating other holistic practices with Ayurveda offers a comprehensive and personalized approach to healing that addresses the interconnectedness of mind, body, and spirit. By combining the ancient wisdom of Ayurveda with complementary healing modalities from around the world, individuals can access a diverse toolkit of approaches to support their journey towards optimal health and well-being. Whether through yoga, massage therapy, energy healing, nutritional therapy, herbal medicine, mind-body practices, or spiritual practices, integrating other holistic practices with Ayurveda allows individuals to cultivate greater awareness, balance, and vitality in their lives.

Building a Comprehensive Wellness Plan

In today's fast-paced world, achieving and maintaining optimal health requires a multifaceted approach that addresses the complex interplay of physical, mental, emotional, and spiritual factors. Building a comprehensive wellness plan that integrates the ancient wisdom of Ayurveda with other complementary healing practices offers a holistic framework for promoting health and well-being in modern living. By combining the strengths of Ayurveda with other holistic modalities, individuals can create a personalized roadmap to vibrant health and vitality that honors their unique constitution, lifestyle, and goals.

1. **Assessment and Evaluation**: The first step in building a comprehensive wellness plan is to conduct a thorough assessment of your current health status, lifestyle habits, and wellness goals. This may involve consulting with healthcare providers from various disciplines, including Ayurvedic practitioners, allopathic physicians, nutritionists, and other holistic practitioners. Through physical exams, diagnostic tests, and in-depth consultations, healthcare providers can gain a comprehensive understanding of your unique needs and develop a tailored plan to support your health and well-being.
2. **Incorporating Ayurvedic Principles**: Ayurveda provides a foundational framework for understanding health and wellness based on the principles of balance, harmony, and holistic living. Incorporating Ayurvedic principles into your wellness plan involves

identifying your unique mind-body constitution (dosha), understanding the influence of the doshas on your health, and implementing lifestyle practices, dietary guidelines, and herbal remedies that support balance and vitality. By aligning your daily routines, dietary choices, and self-care practices with Ayurvedic wisdom, you can promote optimal health and prevent imbalances before they manifest as disease.

3. **Integrating Holistic Modalities**: Building a comprehensive wellness plan involves integrating other holistic modalities that complement Ayurveda and address various aspects of health and well-being. This may include incorporating practices such as yoga, meditation, massage therapy, energy healing, nutritional therapy, herbal medicine, mind-body practices, and spiritual practices into your daily routine. By combining these modalities with Ayurveda, you can access a diverse toolkit of approaches to support your physical, mental, emotional, and spiritual health.

4. **Setting Realistic Goals**: Setting realistic and achievable goals is essential for success in any wellness plan. Work with your healthcare providers to establish clear, measurable goals that align with your values, priorities, and lifestyle. Whether your goals involve improving your diet, increasing physical activity, managing stress, or cultivating mindfulness, breaking them down into smaller, manageable steps can make them more attainable and sustainable over the long term.

5. **Creating a Customized Action Plan**: Once you've identified your goals, work with your healthcare providers to create a customized action plan that outlines the specific steps you'll take to achieve them. This may involve implementing dietary changes, establishing a regular exercise routine, incorporating stress management techniques, scheduling regular check-ins with your healthcare team, and tracking your progress over time. By taking a proactive and systematic approach to your wellness plan, you can stay focused, motivated, and accountable to your health goals.

6. **Monitoring and Adjusting**: Building a comprehensive wellness plan is an ongoing process that requires continuous monitoring and adjustment. Stay attuned to your body's signals, track your progress towards your goals, and be open to making changes as needed along the way. Regularly reassess your health status, reevaluate your priorities, and adjust your action plan accordingly to ensure

that it remains relevant and effective in supporting your evolving needs and goals.
7. **Cultivating Self-Care Practices**: Self-care is an essential component of any wellness plan and involves nurturing your physical, mental, emotional, and spiritual well-being on a daily basis. Incorporate self-care practices such as mindfulness, relaxation techniques, creative expression, and time in nature into your daily routine to promote balance, resilience, and overall well-being. By prioritizing self-care and making time for activities that nourish and rejuvenate you, you can sustain your health and vitality over the long term.
8. **Seeking Support and Accountability**: Building a comprehensive wellness plan can be challenging, and it's essential to seek support and accountability from your healthcare team, friends, family, and community. Surround yourself with people who share your commitment to health and well-being, and lean on them for encouragement, motivation, and guidance along the way. Regularly connect with your healthcare providers for support, feedback, and adjustments to your plan as needed to ensure that you stay on track towards your health goals.

In conclusion, building a comprehensive wellness plan that integrates Ayurveda with other holistic practices offers a powerful approach to promoting health and well-being in modern living. By incorporating Ayurvedic principles, integrating complementary healing modalities, setting realistic goals, creating a customized action plan, monitoring and adjusting as needed, cultivating self-care practices, and seeking support and accountability, you can create a roadmap to vibrant health and vitality that honors your unique needs and aspirations. Embrace the journey of self-discovery and empowerment as you embark on the path towards holistic wellness, and trust in the wisdom of Ayurveda and other holistic practices to guide you towards a life of balance, harmony, and vitality.

Conclusion: Embracing Ayurveda

Sustaining Your Ayurvedic Lifestyle

As we reach the culmination of our exploration into Ayurveda, it becomes evident that this ancient wisdom offers a profound blueprint for navigating the complexities of modern living with grace, balance, and vitality. Throughout this journey, we've delved into the timeless principles of Ayurveda, explored its practical applications in daily life, and discovered how it can be integrated with other holistic practices to create a comprehensive approach to health and well-being. Now, as we conclude our exploration, it's time to reflect on how we can sustain our Ayurvedic lifestyle and continue reaping its benefits in the long term.

1. **Cultivating Mindfulness and Awareness**: At the heart of Ayurveda lies the practice of mindfulness and awareness - the ability to stay present, attuned to our body's signals, and responsive to its needs. Sustaining an Ayurvedic lifestyle requires cultivating this quality of mindfulness in all aspects of our lives, from our dietary choices and daily routines to our thoughts, emotions, and interactions with others. By staying connected to our inner wisdom and intuition, we can make choices that support our health and well-being on a moment-to-moment basis.
2. **Honoring Seasonal Rhythms**: Ayurveda teaches us to live in harmony with the rhythms of nature, honoring the cyclical changes of the seasons and adjusting our lifestyle accordingly. Sustaining an Ayurvedic lifestyle involves attuning ourselves to the qualities of each season - the heat of summer, the cold of winter, the dampness of spring, and the dryness of fall - and making appropriate adjustments to our diet, daily routine, and self-care practices. By aligning ourselves with the seasonal rhythms, we can support our body's natural healing processes and promote balance and vitality year-round.
3. **Nurturing Self-Care Practices**: Self-care is an essential aspect of sustaining an Ayurvedic lifestyle and involves nurturing our physical, mental, emotional, and spiritual well-being on a daily basis. This may include practices such as yoga, meditation, massage, herbal therapies, and time spent in nature, as well as

simple acts of self-kindness and compassion. By prioritizing self-care and making time for activities that nourish and rejuvenate us, we can sustain our health and vitality over the long term.
4. **Maintaining Balance and Harmony**: Ayurveda teaches us that health is a dynamic state of balance and harmony that requires continuous attention and adjustment. Sustaining an Ayurvedic lifestyle involves staying attuned to the fluctuations of our mind, body, and spirit and making conscious choices to restore balance whenever imbalances arise. This may involve adjusting our diet, lifestyle, and self-care practices, seeking support from healthcare providers, and practicing self-reflection and introspection to identify the root causes of imbalance.
5. **Seeking Support and Community**: Sustaining an Ayurvedic lifestyle is not a solitary journey but rather a collective endeavor that benefits from the support and guidance of others. Seek out community, whether it be through local Ayurvedic practitioners, wellness centers, online forums, or social groups, where you can connect with like-minded individuals, share experiences and insights, and support each other on your journey towards holistic health and well-being.
6. **Remaining Open to Growth and Evolution**: Finally, sustaining an Ayurvedic lifestyle requires an attitude of openness, curiosity, and willingness to embrace growth and evolution. Ayurveda is a living, breathing tradition that has evolved over thousands of years, and its principles continue to resonate and adapt to the changing needs of modern society. Remain open to new insights, discoveries, and practices that deepen your understanding of Ayurveda and support your journey towards greater health, vitality, and fulfillment.

In conclusion, sustaining an Ayurvedic lifestyle is a journey of self-discovery, empowerment, and transformation that requires dedication, commitment, and ongoing practice. By cultivating mindfulness and awareness, honoring seasonal rhythms, nurturing self-care practices, maintaining balance and harmony, seeking support and community, and remaining open to growth and evolution, we can sustain our Ayurvedic lifestyle and continue reaping its benefits in all aspects of our lives. Embrace the wisdom of Ayurveda as a guiding light on your journey towards holistic health and well-being, and trust in its timeless principles to support you in living a life of balance, vitality, and joy.

Continuing Education and Resources

As we come to the end of our journey into the world of Ayurveda, it's important to recognize that the path of learning and growth is never-ending. Embracing Ayurveda is not just about adopting a set of practices or principles; it's about committing to a lifelong journey of self-discovery, empowerment, and transformation. In this concluding chapter, we'll explore the importance of continuing education and highlight resources that can support you on your Ayurvedic journey.

1. **The Importance of Continuing Education**: Ayurveda is a vast and multifaceted science that encompasses a wide range of principles, practices, and philosophies. As you continue to deepen your understanding of Ayurveda, it's essential to remain open to new insights, perspectives, and discoveries. Continuing education allows you to expand your knowledge, refine your skills, and stay connected to the evolving landscape of Ayurvedic healing. Whether through formal education programs, workshops, seminars, or self-study, ongoing learning enriches your Ayurvedic journey and empowers you to integrate Ayurvedic principles into all aspects of your life.
2. **Advanced Studies and Specializations**: For those who are passionate about delving deeper into Ayurveda, advanced studies and specializations offer opportunities to explore specialized areas of interest in greater depth. Advanced training programs, mentorship opportunities, and clinical internships provide hands-on experience and guidance from experienced practitioners, allowing you to refine your skills and deepen your understanding of Ayurvedic principles and practices. Whether you're interested in herbal medicine, clinical Ayurveda, Ayurvedic psychology, or another specialized area, advanced studies can help you become a more skilled and effective practitioner.
3. **Professional Associations and Organizations**: Professional associations and organizations play a vital role in supporting the Ayurvedic community and providing resources for practitioners and enthusiasts alike. Joining a professional association allows you

to connect with like-minded individuals, access continuing education opportunities, and stay informed about developments in the field. Additionally, many professional associations offer certification programs, networking events, and other resources to support your professional development and growth as an Ayurvedic practitioner.

4. **Books, Journals, and Publications**: Books, journals, and publications are valuable resources for deepening your understanding of Ayurveda and staying informed about current research, trends, and practices. There are countless books available on Ayurvedic principles, diet and nutrition, herbal medicine, lifestyle practices, and more, written by esteemed authors and experts in the field. Journals and publications provide access to peer-reviewed research articles, case studies, and clinical insights that can inform your practice and enhance your knowledge base.

5. **Online Courses and Webinars**: In today's digital age, online courses and webinars offer convenient and accessible ways to learn about Ayurveda from the comfort of your own home. Many reputable institutions and organizations offer online courses on a wide range of topics, including Ayurvedic principles, diet and nutrition, herbal medicine, yoga, meditation, and more. Webinars provide opportunities to engage with experts, ask questions, and deepen your understanding of specific topics through live or recorded presentations.

6. **Community and Support Groups**: Building connections with others who share your passion for Ayurveda can provide invaluable support, inspiration, and camaraderie on your journey. Whether through local meetups, online forums, social media groups, or retreats and conferences, connecting with fellow Ayurvedic enthusiasts allows you to share experiences, exchange ideas, and learn from one another's insights and perspectives. Community and support groups offer a sense of belonging and encouragement as you navigate the ups and downs of your Ayurvedic journey.

7. **Personal Practice and Self-Care**: Ultimately, the most important resource on your Ayurvedic journey is your own personal practice and self-care. Cultivating a daily routine that includes Ayurvedic practices such as dinacharya (daily routine), sattvic diet, yoga, meditation, and self-reflection allows you to embody the principles of Ayurveda in your own life and experience their transformative power firsthand. Prioritize your own health

and well-being, listen to your body's wisdom, and trust in the guidance of Ayurveda to support you on your path towards holistic health and vitality.

In conclusion, embracing Ayurveda is a lifelong journey of learning, growth, and self-discovery. By committing to continuing education, staying connected to resources and community, and prioritizing your own self-care and personal practice, you can sustain and deepen your Ayurvedic lifestyle for years to come. Remember that Ayurveda is not just a system of healing; it's a way of life that offers profound insights into the interconnectedness of mind, body, and spirit. Embrace Ayurveda as a guiding light on your journey towards holistic health, and trust in its wisdom to support you in living a life of balance, vitality, and joy.

Community and Support

As we reach the conclusion of our journey into the world of Ayurveda, it becomes evident that community and support play a vital role in sustaining and enriching our Ayurvedic lifestyle. Throughout this book, we have explored the ancient wisdom of Ayurveda, delved into its practical applications in daily life, and discovered how it can empower us to thrive in the modern world. Now, as we conclude our exploration, let us reflect on the importance of community and support in our Ayurvedic journey.

1. **Finding Your Tribe**: Embracing Ayurveda is not just about adopting a set of practices or principles; it's about connecting with a community of like-minded individuals who share your passion for holistic health and well-being. Whether through local meetups, online forums, social media groups, or Ayurvedic retreats and workshops, finding your tribe allows you to connect with others who are on a similar path and share experiences, insights, and support along the way.
2. **Sharing Experiences and Insights**: Community provides a platform for sharing experiences, insights, and wisdom gained from our Ayurvedic journey. By sharing our challenges, triumphs, and learnings with others, we can offer support and encouragement to one another and inspire each other to stay committed to our health and well-being goals. Whether through in-person gatherings, virtual discussions, or written reflections, sharing our experiences strengthens the bonds of community and fosters a sense of connection and belonging.
3. **Accessing Resources and Guidance**: Community offers access to a wealth of resources, guidance, and expertise that can support us on our Ayurvedic journey. Whether through local Ayurvedic practitioners, wellness centers, or online communities, connecting with knowledgeable individuals allows us to access information, ask questions, and seek guidance on specific health concerns or Ayurvedic practices. By tapping into the collective wisdom of the community, we can enrich our understanding of Ayurveda and enhance our ability to integrate its principles into our lives.
4. **Accountability and Motivation**: Community provides accountability and motivation to stay committed to our Ayurvedic

lifestyle. By sharing our goals, intentions, and progress with others, we can hold ourselves accountable to our commitments and stay motivated to prioritize our health and well-being. Whether through accountability partners, support groups, or wellness challenges, community provides a framework for setting goals, tracking progress, and celebrating successes together.
5. **Cultivating Connection and Belonging**: Perhaps most importantly, community fosters a sense of connection and belonging that nourishes the soul and supports our overall well-being. In a world that can often feel fragmented and disconnected, finding a community of like-minded individuals allows us to experience a sense of belonging and unity that is deeply fulfilling and enriching. By coming together in shared purpose and intention, we create a space where we can authentically be ourselves, support one another, and co-create a world that reflects our values and aspirations.

In conclusion, embracing Ayurveda is not just a personal journey; it's a collective endeavor that thrives on community and support. By connecting with others who share our passion for holistic health and well-being, we create a space where we can learn, grow, and evolve together. Whether through local gatherings, online communities, or shared experiences, community provides a framework for sharing wisdom, offering support, and cultivating connection and belonging. As we continue on our Ayurvedic journey, let us remember the importance of community and support in sustaining and enriching our path towards health, vitality, and wholeness.